W9-ATX-465

The Sinus Handbook
A Self-Help Guide

by

Muriel MacFarlane, RN, MA

United Research Publishers

Published by United Research Publishers

Printed and bound in the United States of America

ISBN 1-887053-08-5

Library of Congress Catalog Card number 96-61828

Copyright © 1997

The information in this book is not intended to replace the advice of your physician. You should consult your doctor regarding any medical condition which concerns you. The material presented in this book is intended to inform and educate the reader with a view to making some intelligent choices in pursuing the goal of living your life in a healthy, vigorous manner. Neither the author nor the publisher assumes any responsibility or liability for the judgements or decisions any reader might make as a result of reading this publication.

Book design by The Final Draft, Encinitas, CA

Cover design by The Art Department, Encinitas, CA

Order additional copies from:

United Research Publishers
P.O. Box 232344
Encinitas, CA 92023-2344

Full 90-day money back guarantee if not satisfied.

CONTENTS

Introduction 1

Section I 3

   The Functions of the Sinuses 4

   The Nose 8

      The Sense of Smell 13

      The Sense of Taste 15

   The Pharynx 16

      Nasopharynx 18

      Oropharynx 18

      Laryngopharynx 18

   Larynx 19

      Laryngitis 21

   Ears 22

      Acute Otitis Media 22

      Swimmer's Ear 30

   Your Immune System 31

      The Thymus Gland 35

      Acid/Alkaline Balance 36

   Colds and Flu 37

      The Common Cold 38

      The Flu 39

Section II 41

   Causes of Sinusitis 42

   Diagnosing Sinusitis 44

      Angioedema (allergic localized swelling) 45

      Cellulitis 45

      Headache 46

      Neuralgia of the trigeminal nerve 46

      Temporal arteritis 46

      Toothache 46

      Tumors 47

The Goal of Treatment 47
Tracking Down the Start of the Problem 48
    The Common Culprit 49
    Irritants 50
    Pollutants 61
    The Effects of Cold Air 63
    The Effects of Dry Air 64
    Allergy 66
    Hazardous Occupations 74
    Contributing Physical Factors 75
Symptoms of Sinusitis 76
    Colds 77
    Bronchitis 78
    Sinusitis 79
Diagnosing Chronic Sinusitis 85
    Acute Sinusitis 88
    Chronic Sinusitis 90
The Number One Health Problem in the U.S. 91
    Asthma 92
    Allergic Rhinitis 106
    Bronchitis 109
    Major Contributory Factors 111

Section III **119**

Treating Sinusitis 119
    Antibiotics 121
    Decongestants 128
    Decongestant Nasal Sprays 129
    Antihistamines 130
    Antitussives (cough suppressants) 132
    Analgesics (pain relievers) 132
    Hydration 133
    Saline Spray and Irrigation 134
    Otolaryngology Evaluation 138
    Surgery 140

Treating Asthma 141
    Diagnosis 147
    Treatment 150
Treating Allergy 164
Treating Bronchitis 178
    Acute Bronchitis 178
    Chronic Bronchitis 178
    Sinobronchitis 180
    Chronic Obstructive Bronchitis 182

Section IV **185**
Are You Ready for Healthy Sinuses? 185
The Inner Environment—
       Building an Optimum Immune System 187
    Hygiene 188
    Alcohol-Nicotine-Caffeine 190
    Stop That Cold in its First Stages 193
    Rest to Repair 194
    Sleep 195
    Antioxidants—the Green Pastures of Life 201
    Herbs—Concentrated Food 205
    Phytochemicals—Immune System Enhancers 207
    Diet—For Overall Health 209
    Exercise 214
    Consider Allergy 214
    Water—the Essential Nutrient 216
    Rest—the Ease Restorer 218
    Stress—the Killer "Virus" 221
    Stress Management 223
Avoidance of Triggers 225
    Dust 226
    Dust Mites 227
    Cockroaches 228
    Cats and Dogs 228
    Mold 229

Pollen 230
A Healthy Indoor Environment 231
   Negative Ions 233
   Household Plants 234
   Radon 234
Candida Albicans—Something to Consider 235
Folk Remedies—You Might Want to Try 239
   Honey 240
   Lemon peel 240
   Fenugreek 240
   Ginkgo biloba 240
   Ice 241
   Salt water 241
   Steam 241
   Aromatherapy 242
   Hot beverages 242
   Nose blowing 242
   Spicy foods 242
   Coughing 243
   Fatigue 243
   Headache 244
   Runny nose 244
   Sore throat 244
   Stuffy nose 244
   Wheezing 245
Thymus
   A Long Ignored Part of the Immune System 245
A Few Additional Helpful Hints 246

Section V **249**

The Search for Perfect Health 249
   Holistic Medicine 251
   Biofeedback 255
   Yoga 256
   Hypnotherapy 257

Cognitive Therapy 258
Guided Imagery and Visualization 258
Osteopathic Medicine 261
Chiropractic 262
Naturopathic Medicine 262
Meditation 263
Body Work 264
Peace of Mind 266
Faith and Healing...................................... 268
Acupressure and Acupuncture 272
Ayurveda 275
Traditional Chinese Medicine 276
Herbalism 278
Homeopathy 281
Flower Essences...................................... 285
Aromatherapy and the Use of Essential Oils 287
Reflexology 289

Bibliography 293

Index 299

Introduction

One out of every seven Americans complains at some time or another about the condition of his or her sinuses. Everyone has heard someone say they are suffering from a "sinus headache" and, unfortunately, most of us can nod our heads in understanding and sympathy. We know exactly the feeling they mean. The unhappy condition of the American sinuses may be the most common ailment, surpassing the even common cold, as a reason to consult a physician.

Most people think of the sinuses as two small spots somewhere inside the head, right behind the forehead and above the eyes, as the location of their misery. You know it when you are suffering from a head cold, your head is aching, your nose is all stuffed up; that spot, right above your eyes, seems to be where most of the trouble is centered.

Pressure above the eyes during the day, a headache that may prevent you from working, the drip of fluid down the throat during the night and often lots of nasty looking thick yellow mucus from the nose. Not a pretty sight to see or have others see, and not a pretty thought, to experience a sinus condition, or to dread having one—again.

Clearly sinusitis is a condition that is not a lot of fun, doesn't get much sympathy, and never adds anything to your good looks, with lots of tired and soggy tissues sticking out of all your available pockets.

In order to have a clear understanding of just what happens when the sinuses cause suffering—from recurring colds, allergy, polyps or other causes, with the resulting headache, pain or constant drainage—it is necessary to know what these structures look like, what they do, and how they function in the body.

Section I

The word sinus actually means "a hollow space" and we have a great number of them throughout the body. There are sinuses of the eye, the heart, the kidney, the rectum; they are located throughout the entire body.

However, when we speak of our aching sinuses, most people are referring to the ones located in the bones of the face and head that surround and connect the nasal cavities. These hollow, air-filled spaces are lined with the same membrane that lines the nose, as well as the same vascular and nerve supply; these sinuses, or hollow spaces, drain into the nose cavity through openings in the skull called *ostia*.

Ostia are thin ducts, no larger than the lead in a pencil. On average, they are approximately two millimeters in diameter. It is easy to understand that it doesn't take a lot to block such a small tube. The ducts of the maxillary sinuses are located at the top of those sinuses, making drainage difficult. A series of small ducts in the nasal wall drain the ethmoid sinuses, and they too, are easily blocked. Evolution has not been kind to man when it comes to the sinuses. They would drain more readily if we walked on all fours instead of upright. But, we're stuck with our upright posture and the resultant drainage difficulties that posture causes.

The Functions of the Sinuses

The sinuses of the head have seven main functions:

1. They lighten the weight of the skull. The hollow spaces in the bones of the head reduce the weight of the head, so that the head isn't too heavy to carry around all day on top of the slender structure of the neck.

2. They act as resonating chambers for the voice, to give it timbre and character. Genetics dictate the shape and the structure of the skull and consequently the shape and size of the sinuses. This, along with the structure of the vocal cords and other body parts involved in the production of speech, determines the sound of the speaking voice. When some-

one has a head cold it is not just the irritated throat that makes the voice sound different, it is also the muffled resonance of that voice through the now mucus-filled sinuses.

3. They warm the air as we breathe.

4. They humidify the air we breathe.

5. They act as a cushion, a buffer for the interior of the skull. If we are injured, they buffer any blow to the brain, working something like an air bag in an automobile.

6. Filled with air, they act as insulators, to keep the base of the brain, which is very near to the inside of the nose, warm.

7. Along with the nose, they serve as the body's chief protector of the lungs. This function is performed by acting as a filter: defending against bacteria, viruses, dirt and dust, pollen and anything else airborne that could cause harm to the lungs and the respiratory system. Being able to breathe is primary to staying alive, and these magnificent structures— which we often ignore or get angry with

because they cause us pain—play a primary role in the defense of our health and our ability to breathe.

There are four sinuses in the skull: the maxillary, the ethmoid, the frontal and the sphenoid. They are known collectively as the *paranasal sinuses* and are named for the bone(s) of the skull in which they are located.

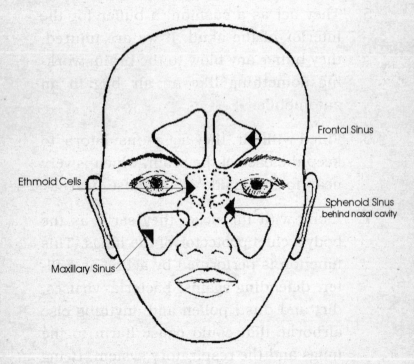

Frontal Sinus

Ethmoid Cells

Sphenoid Sinus
behind nasal cavity

Maxillary Sinus

1. The frontal bone forms the forehead, the upper portion of the eye sockets and most of the anterior (front) part of the

cranial floor. The frontal sinuses are above the eyes, just above the nose and directly behind the forehead, and only appear after the second year of life.

2. The maxillary bones form the upper jaw. The maxillary sinuses are the largest and are pyramid-shaped hollow spaces located inside each cheekbone. They are present at birth. They enlarge gradually until puberty and rapidly thereafter, and reach their full size sometime between the ages of sixteen to twenty-one.

3. The ethmoid bone helps form a portion of the cranial floor, the inside walls of the eye sockets, the upper portions of the nasal septum and most of the side walls of the nasal roof. It is the principal supporting structure of the nasal cavity. The ethmoid sinuses consist of a series of small cavities known as *ethmoid cells* which can range in number from three to eighteen. At birth they are mere slits or grooves in the bone, enlarging gradually through puberty. They are behind the maxillaries and between the bony orbits of the eye. They are

actually complex networks of small air pockets.

4. The sphenoid bone is located at the base of the skull and is known as the "keystone" of the cranial floor because it binds the other cranial bones together. The sphenoid sinuses are deep within the skull behind the nose.

Secretions from these sinuses drain into the nasal cavity through quite small tubes or ducts. An inflammation of the membranes due to an allergic reaction or an infection is known as *sinusitis*. If these membranes swell sufficiently, they can block drainage into the nasal cavity; fluid pressure then builds up in the paranasal sinuses and results in a common sinus headache.

The Nose

The nose has an external portion jutting out from the face as well as an internal portion which lies hidden inside the skull. Externally, the nose consists of a supporting framework of bone and cartilage covered with skin. The bridge of the nose is formed by the nasal bones, which hold it in a fixed position. Because it has a framework of pliable cartilage, the rest of the external nose is quite flexible. On the underside of the external nose are two openings called the *nostrils* or *external nares.*

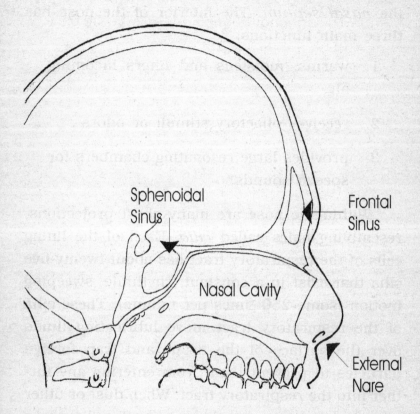

Sphenoidal Sinus

Frontal Sinus

Nasal Cavity

External Nare

The internal region of the nose is a large cavity within the skull, below the cranium and above the mouth. The internal nose merges with the external nose. To the rear it communicates with the throat through two openings known as the *internal nares.* The four sinuses and the nasolacrimal (nasal-tear) ducts open into the internal nose.

9

The inside of the nose is divided into right and left *nasal cavities* by a vertical wall known as the *nasal septum*. The interior of the nose has three main functions:

1. warms, moistens and filters incoming air.

2. receives olfactory stimuli or odors

3. provides large resonating chambers for speech sounds.

Within the nose are many short projections, resembling hairs called *cilia.* Each of the lining cells of the respiratory tract has about twenty-five cilia that exist in a constant, rhythmic, sweeping motion (some 250 times per minute). These cilia of the respiratory tract move lubricating fluids over the surface of the tissue and trap foreign particles to prevent them from entering any further into the respiratory tract. When dust or other particles are trapped in this mucus, the cilia sweep them toward the back of the nose, where they go down the throat and are broken down by stomach acids for excretion. These small hairlike projections work constantly, beating with a regular rhythm in their effort to sweep the dust-laden mucus onward, and can be damaged by excess heat, such as the heated air inhaled in cigarette smoking.

When air enters the nostrils, it passes into the first portion of the nose, the vestibule. This vestibule is lined with a mucous membrane covered with coarse hairs that filter out large dust particles. The air then passes into the rest of the nasal cavity. Inside this next portion there are three shelves known as turbinates which extend out from the back wall of this cavity. Mucous membranes line the cavity and its shelves. The olfactory or smell receptors lie in the membrane lining the upper portion. Below this, the membrane contains many small goblet cells which secrete mucus. (They are called goblet cells because the mucus accumulates in the upper half of the cells, causing the area to bulge out. The whole cell resembles a goblet or wine glass.) Mucus from this tissue serves as a lubricant that prevents friction. Here there are also cilia and capillaries. As the air whirls around the turbinates, it is warmed by these capillaries, and mucus from the goblet cells moistens the air and traps more and even smaller dust particles. The cilia move the resulting mucus-dust packages along to the throat so that they can be eliminated from the body.

As air passes through the top of the cavity, chemicals in the air may stimulate the olfactory receptors.

The sinuses perform a valuable act by humidifying dry air that would irritate the lungs, and regulating the temperature of the incoming air. Cooling excessively hot air and warming extremely cold air that would shock the lungs: this is a function essential to life. Humans inhale thousands of times a day, moving approximately two gallons of air per minute or three thousand gallons per day through our noses. The nose and the sinuses are constantly at work shielding the essential lungs from harm.

One-of-a kind tissue, the respiratory epithelium, lines the sinuses, the nose and the lungs. All three are part of the respiratory tract, which performs that most essential function necessary to continue life: breathing. There is a continuous mucous membrane lining the sinuses, all the ducts and the nasal passages. If anything causes this lining in the nose to swell, it also affects the same tissue in the ducts and the sinuses. Swelling can cause the passageways to narrow and limit the work of the cilia, which are attempting to sweep all dust laden mucus along constantly.

The mucous membrane and its hard-working hairlike projections, the cilia, are a defense mechanism against infections and all other foreign matter that could enter the respiratory system through the nose. The mucus covering the maxillary sinus is ordinarily entirely cleared every ten minutes, and the mucous membrane that lines the entire respiratory tract produces between a pint and a quart of mucus daily.

We should all be in awe of the work this system performs, and most of the time, performs so well.

The Sense of Smell

The total area of olfactory tissue in the interior of the nose is only about 0.4 square inches on each side. It includes the inside wall of the turbinate (dividing wall) and the back surface of the septum. It consists of a network of supporting cells and olfactory receptor cells. Cilia project from the top of these cells into the mucous membrane of the nose. At one end of each cell, a small central core of a nerve projects upward with millions of other olfactory nerves to the olfactory bulb, where they continue in nerve tracts to the smell-sensing areas of the brain. There is an interrelationship between the sensation of smell and taste, and most people complain of impaired sense of taste when they have any nasal congestion.

The sensation of smell depends on the diffusion of inhaled air into the still air of the upper portion of the nasal cavity. Sniffing causes the nostrils to dilate and the direction of the forward part of the nose to be altered so that the stream of the inhaled air is directed toward these smell receptors. Odors can be perceived in very minute quantities and can be very finely discriminated, providing, of course, that there is not blockage of the nasal passages.

Just how these receptors are stimulated and how discrimination between odors is achieved is not completely understood. It is generally thought that substances detected by smell are usually soluble in fat. Since the membrane of an olfactory hair is largely fat, it is assumed that molecules of substances to be smelled are dissolved in the membrane where they initiate the nerve impulse. The sensation of smell happens quickly, but adaptation to odors also occurs rapidly. For this reason, we become accustomed to some odors and are also able to endure unpleasant ones. Receptors in the brain appear to be stimulated by memory and to form a myriad of associations very readily. Attempts to classify odors has not been very successful, since there is not one kind of receptor for each kind of odor. It appears that we are able to distinguish among the several thousand odors as a result of some sort of a mixing process, such as occurs in color perception. One classification attempt, based on similarities of molecular structure and odor, names the following as seven primary classes of odors: camphoraceous, musky, floral, pepperminty, ethereal, pungent and putrid.

The supporting cells of the nasal epithelium and tear ducts are supplied by branches of the facial nerves, the same ones that receive stimuli of pain, cold, heat, tickling and pressure. Anything that causes the mucous membranes of the interior of the nose and the sinuses to overproduce mucus, such as an infection or an allergen, will interfere with the proper functioning of the olfactory structures, with a resultant decrease in the ability to smell.

Many people might think that the loss of the sense of smell is unimportant. In addition to its effect on the sense of taste, where it is a very important part of stimulating the appetite and helping us know whether or not food is safe to eat, the ability to smell is a very important protective mechanism, giving us first warning of a variety of dangers—including fire or harmful chemicals.

The Sense of Taste

The receptors for sensations of taste are located in the taste buds. These buds are most numerous on the tongue, but they are also found on the soft palate and in the throat. In order for these cells to be stimulated, the substances we taste must be in solution in the saliva so that they can enter the taste pores in the taste buds. Despite the many substances we taste, there are basically only four taste sensations: sour, salt, bitter and sweet. The subtle differences in taste are controlled by the sense of smell, rather than taste, and the desire for food may decrease if the sense of smell is diminished. Taste is another important protective mechanism. Coupled with the sense of smell, it is a defense against spoiled or unsavory foods, which might be dangerous to eat.

Anything that causes the mucous membranes of the interior of the nose and the sinuses to over-produce mucus (such as sinusitis) will interfere with the proper functioning of the olfactory structures, contributing to the decrease in the ability to interpret tastes.

The Pharynx

The pharynx, or throat, is a tube about 5 inches long that starts at the internal nares and runs part way down the neck.

The pharynx lies just back of the nasal cavity and mouth, and just in front of the vertebrae of the spine. Its walls are composed of skeletal muscles. The interior of these walls are lined with mucous membranes. This structurally simple tube serves as a passage way for air and food, and provides a resonating chamber for speech sounds. This mucous membrane-lined muscular tube contains largely voluntary muscle. Swallowing is a consciously initiated act rather than a reflex. However, once begun, reflexive mechanisms propel food down the esophagus to the stomach.

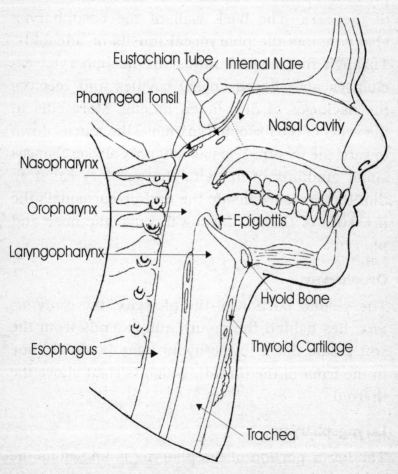

Nasopharynx

The uppermost portion of the pharynx is known as the *nasopharynx.* This part lies behind the nose and extends down to the soft palate. There are four openings in its walls: two internal nares plus two openings that lead into the auditory tubes of the ears. The back wall of the nasopharynx also contains the pharyngeal tonsils or adenoids. Through the internal nares the nasopharynx exchanges air with the nasal cavities and receives the packages of dust-laden mucus. More cilia in the walls of the nasopharynx move the mucus down toward the mouth. The nasopharynx also exchanges small amounts of air with the auditory canal so that the pressure inside the middle ear equals the pressure of the air flowing through the nose and pharynx.

Oropharynx

The second portion of the pharynx, the *oropharynx,* lies behind the mouth and extends from the soft palate down to the hyoid bone (a small bone in the front of the throat), which is right above the thyroid.

Laryngopharynx

The lower portion of the pharynx is known as the *laryngopharynx.* It extends downward from the hyoid bone and empties into the esophagus (food tube) in the back and the larynx (voice box) in the front. This section of the pharynx is both respiratory and digestive in function.

Larynx

The *larynx*, or voice box, is a short passageway that connects the pharynx with the trachea, and it lies in the middle of the neck. The trachea is the part of the tube that branches into the bronchi of the lungs. The walls of the larynx are supported by pieces of cartilage. The largest of these, the *thyroid cartilage* or Adam's apple, is larger in males than in females.

The *epiglottis* is a large, leaf-shaped piece of cartilage lying on top of the larynx. The "stem" of the epiglottis is attached to the thyroid cartilage, but the "leaf" portion is unattached and free to move up and down, just like a door on a hinge. In fact, the epiglottis is sometimes known as the "trap door." As the larynx moves upward and forward during swallowing, the free edge of the epiglottis moves downward and forms a cap over the larynx. The larynx is closed off so liquids and foods are routed into the esophagus and kept out of the tache. If anything but air passes into the larynx, a cough reflex tries to expel the material.

Most of us have, at one time or another, said we have "swallowed the wrong way," meaning that something got past the epiglottis and we found ourselves choking and coughing. For some reason or another, usually because we are talking and laughing as we are eating, the timing of the closure of the epiglottis wasn't quite right.

The mucous membrane of the larynx is arranged into two pairs of folds, an upper pair known as the *false vocal folds* and the lower pair known as the *vocal folds* or *true vocal cords.* The air passageway between the folds is known as the *glottis.*

Just below the mucous membrane of the true vocal cords lie bands of elastic cartilage that are stretched between pieces of rigid cartilage, just like the strings on a guitar. Skeletal muscles are attached to the pieces of rigid cartilage and then to the vocal cords themselves. When the muscles contract, they pull the strings of elastic cartilage tight and stretch the cords out into the air passageways so that the glottis is narrowed. If air is directed against the vocal folds, they vibrate and set up sound waves in the column of air in the pharynx, nose, and mouth. The greater the pressure of air, the louder the sound.

Pitch is controlled by the tension on the true vocal cords. If the cords are pulled taut by the muscles, the vibrate more rapidly and a higher pitch results. Lower sounds are produced by decreasing the muscular tension on the cords. Vocal cords are usually thicker and longer in males than in females, and they vibrate more slowly. This is why men have a lower range of pitch than women normally have.

Sound originates from the vibration of the true vocal cords. But other structures are necessary for converting the sound into recognizable speech. For instance, the pharynx, mouth, nasal cavities, and paranasal sinuses all act as resonating chambers that give the voice its human and individual quality. By constricting and relaxing the muscles in the walls of the pharynx we produce the vowel sounds. Muscles of the face, tongue, and lips help us to enunciate the spoken words.

From here, the trachea or windpipe extends down into the bronchi and then to the lungs. The esophagus, which lies behind the trachea, extends downward through the diaphragm and terminates in the upper portion of the stomach.

Laryngitis

Laryngitis is an inflammation of the larynx, most often caused by a respiratory infection or by irritants, such as cigarette smoke. Inflammation of the vocal folds themselves causes hoarseness or loss of voice by interfering with the contraction of the cords or causing them to swell so they cannot vibrate freely. Many long-term smokers acquire a permanent hoarseness from the damage done by chronic inflammation. You may be familiar with the term "whiskey tenor" which denotes a husky voice, caused by the constant irritation of these structures by exposure to alcohol.

Ears

Acute Otitis Media

Acute otitis media is a bacterial or viral infection in the middle ear, usually secondary to an upper respiratory infection. It can occur at any age; it is most common in young children, particularly from age three months to three years. Microorganisms may migrate from the nasopharynx to the middle ear over the surface of the Eustachian tube's mucous membrane.

Ear infections are responsible for more visits to the doctor by children under fifteen years old than any other ailment. According to Barton Schmitt, director of general pediatric consultations at Children's Hospital, Denver, an ear infection is the most prevalent complication of a cold in children.

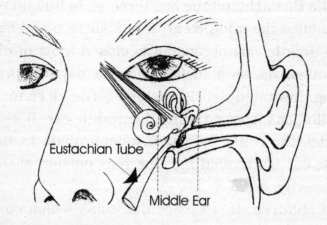

Eustachian Tube

Middle Ear

The Eustachian tube connects the middle ear to the back of the nose. The middle ear and the Eustachian tube are both lined with a membrane very similar to that of the nose, with mucus-producing glands and cilia to sweep the mucus and its trapped debris from the middle ear, through the Eustachian tube, and out into the back portion of the naval cavity. Abnormal Eustachian tube function is the root cause of recurring ear infections. This tube is closed most of the time and it opens only briefly during swallowing, yawning, sniffing and activities associated with straining. When it does open, air passes into and out of the middle ear, fluid is swept (by cilia) from the middle ear into the nose, and then the tube quickly closes again.

The Eustachian tube has three main functions: it ventilates the middle ear; it lets air into and out of the middle ear; because it is closed most of the time, it serves as a highly effective barrier, preventing unwanted debris such as germs, irritants, and allergens from entering the middle ear. It also provides the route by which mucus made in the middle ear is expelled into the rear portion of the nasal cavity.

In children, this Eustachian tube, which connects the nose and the sinuses to the back of the nose and throat, is more or less horizontal. It is not until later in life that it lies in a more downward position, allowing mucus to drain. Since this Eustachian tube does not function the way an adult's does, it doesn't act as an efficient barrier to injurious agents and doesn't permit the ciliary mechanism to clear the ear as well. The child's ear can be easily infected and trap excessive fluid. As the child matures, so does the Eustachian tube. As it grows, it gets better support from its surrounding tissue and bone. This maturation occurs between ages three to six. Beyond six, middle ear infections are much less common in children.

Everyone who has ever flown on an airplane has had the experience of pressure within the ear building up and causing an uncomfortable feeling. This pressure is in the Eustachian tube, which is made up partly of bone and partly of cartilage and is lined with the same cilia and mucous membrane as the sinuses. Adults are advised to chew gum or yawn to alter this pressure within the ear. You have probably heard a young child crying loudly as these pressure changes are greatest—when the plane is losing or gaining altitude—and the baby has no way to relieve this pressure within the ear.

A product available at any pharmacy, known as Earplanes, is available for both adults and children. These Earplanes are inserted into the ear before any flight and are advertised as preventing this pressure buildup. For those with sinus conditions, colds or nasal congestion, who must fly, these might be worthwhile.

Middle ear infections are the most common illness in children seen in emergency rooms or in the pediatrician's office. This condition is quite often seen in conjunction with sinusitis. The bacteria most often responsible for this condition are the same ones responsible for sinus infections.

When a child has otitis media, sinusitis might go unrecognized. These children usually have a persistent, severe earache, with fever up to 105°F, accompanied by nausea, vomiting and diarrhea. Babies often tug or pull on their ears and children who are old enough to talk complain of an earache, and usually do not differentiate the pain in the sinuses from the ear.

Treatment with antibiotics, based on culture of the causative agent, usually lasts for approximately two weeks, at which time both the otitis media and any accompanying sinusitis should be cleared up.

Many young children suffer with frequent bouts of otitis media, sometimes as often as four or five times a year; chronic otitis media can result from acute otitis media, resulting sometimes in permanent hearing loss.

Sometimes, after repeated treatment with antibiotics, some children will be referred to an ear, nose and throat specialist, who will perform a surgery in which a tympanostomy tube is placed in the eardrum to improve the drainage from the middle ear.

Some specialists are attempting to evaluate these children for allergies before resorting to this surgery, which is the most common operation for children which requires them to be subjected to general anesthesia.

Talal M. Nsousli, of the Georgetown University School of Medicine, and colleagues report that food allergies underlie many multiple episodes of otitis media in young children. When 104 children with recurrent ear problems were tested for food allergies, eighty-one were found to react to a food they often ate, and seventy got better when they avoided those foods for four months. Sixty-six of those seventy developed middle ear problems within four months of returning to eating those avoided foods.

Before subjecting your child to such surgery, if you suspect that food allergy may be the cause of this recurring condition, you may want to test your child for food allergies. One of the very effective ways to do this is to eliminate the most common allergenic foods, along with any favorite foods your child craves, for five or six days. Milk should head the list, along with chocolate, eggs, wheat, oats, rye and any coloring or preservative-laden food in the diet.

One ear, nose and throat specialist, Dr. Fred Pullen, claims that as many as seventy-five percent of the children referred to him to have tubes inserted in their ears because of chronic ear infections responded so well to the elimination of dairy products from their diets that the surgery was deemed unnecessary.

If your child is suffering from allergies, he or she will probably feel somewhat uncomfortable during the first few days of an allergy test. Help the child cooperate with the food-elimination diet by being patient and supportive. Provide relief for the discomforts with an extra gram of Vitamin C in freshly squeezed fruit juice diluted with fifty percent distilled water one half hour before each meal. By the third or fourth day, you should notice an improvement in symptoms. Tiredness, headaches, runny nose, or stuffiness should be decreasing if allergy is at the root of your child's condition. With a child who is old enough, he or she can begin to understand just how the food is creating the condition.

On the sixth or seventh day, let the child go back to the regular diet, including the suspect foods. If these foods are producing allergic conditions, there should be a noticeable response. Once you have determined that the child is allergic, you can pinpoint the exact food by repeating the same test, only this time with a few foods at a time.

Sometimes the child will feel so much better that he or she will willingly cooperate in removing the foods from the diet. If the child is cooperative and better, be ready to substitute more nutritious or more palatable foods to replace the ones that will be eliminated.

Before subjecting your child to a tympanostomy, it might be well worth the trouble to try an elimination diet to test for allergy-induced ear infections first.

In a study published in the April, 1994 issue of the *Journal of the American Medical Association,* it was concluded that one-third of the tympanostomy surgeries might be questionable, subjecting several hundred thousand children to unnecessary surgeries to have tubes surgically inserted in their ears with no demonstrable advantage. Furthermore, a team of experts led by Harvard pediatrician Lawrence Kleinmann reported that not only did a tympanostomy offer no demonstrated advantage to these hundreds of thousands of children, the operation needlessly placed them at risk of eardrum scarring and partial loss of hearing.

A study published in the *Journal of the American Medical Association* found that children on antibiotics are actually more prone to otitis recurrences than those who take nothing at all.

Researchers at Penn State found preschoolers who suffer repeated ear infections may be late in development of crucial listening skills, and be at risk for early school problems. In a study conducted by the Greater Boston Otitis Media Study Group, it was found that the more ear infections that children suffer before age three, the lower the children's scores will be on later tests of speech, language and intellectual ability. These infections can easily go unrecognized, especially because they generally affect young children who are unable to recognize or tell parents of their discomfort.

In adults with otitis media, the regular use of a decongestant for a period longer than the usual ten days to two weeks of treatment with the antibiotic is recommended, because adults often complain of a continued decrease in their ability to hear, or that sounds continue to be muffled, after the infection has been treated.

Swimmer's Ear

While water sports can be fun, overexposure to water, wind, and cold can result in an ear problem known as swimmer's ear. The trouble occurs when dead skin or wax collects inside the ear. When this debris gets wet, it can become chapped and swollen and prone to bacterial and fungal problems.

Physicians suggest rinsing the ear with rubbing alcohol or a combination of white vinegar and alcohol after swimming.

Surfer's ear, which can result from chronic swimmer's ear, is characterized by the development of bone tumors or bony spurs under the skin in the ear canal.

For children who swim regularly, it is best to be sure that water does not stay in the ears too long, and teach young children to remove water in the ears by leaning over, side to side, after swimming, to drain the water from their ears, thus avoiding the development of bacterial or fungal problems which can lead to otitis media.

Your Immune System

Since the earliest times, both men and animals have been plagued by unseen enemies—parasites, bacteria, viruses—which have continuously sought to enter and ravage the inner world of the body. Against these minute and dangerous living organisms, animals and men have had to develop some means of defense if they were to live. Over the eons of time, there has evolved a mechanism called immunity—a mysterious and complex process that protects men and animals against attacks by these tiny alien invaders.

In the broadest terms, immunity is the essential function by which we maintain our functional integrity against the threat of entry by foreign chemical substances into the body.

Immunity covers the complex of processes concerned with protection against microorganisms and the acquired specific resistance to reinfection that follows infection by such a pathogen. Immunity ensures our survival; it is a complex group of biologic processes that protects the body against foreign invaders; and a process that builds up resistance to these invaders, sometimes thereby preventing that organism from infecting us twice, by learning to recognize its foreign protein.

The general effects of immunity are to neutralize and destroy alien organisms, and then to build up resistance to further attacks.

Whenever the body recognizes the presence of an invading organism or a protein material it cannot identify as a part of itself, the body normally protects itself by developing an immune response.

In the healthy immune system, an immune response involves the development of protective proteins in response to an invasion by foreign and dangerous protein substances.

The protective proteins are called *antibodies* and the foreign proteins are called *antigens.*

In an immune system damaged by pathologic changes, an immune response may occur in response to certain of the body's own proteins— these proteins are known as self-antigens or autoantigens. These pathologic conditions in which the body directs the immune response against itself are called *autoimmune* diseases.

Antigens are chemical substances that are nearly always protein in nature, and are seen by the body as an attacking force. The structures of antigenic microorganisms such as bacteria and viruses are protein, as are almost all the toxins that they manufacture and release.

Antigens are capable of two highly sophisticated functions, both of which may result in the eventual destruction of the antigens by antibodies. One role of antigens is to initiate an immune response, i.e., antigens stimulate the development of antibodies against themselves. The second role of the antigenic substances is to react specifically with those antibodies that they have developed.

Antibodies, sometimes called immune bodies or immunoglobulins, are protective substances composed of protein that can be detected in the blood. These antibodies perform their complex tasks of defending the body by reacting with antigens in several different ways. Sometimes they disarm bacteria and render them harmless by causing them to clump together; or they might coat a bacterium and make it appetizing to phagocytes (cells which eat up bacteria). Antibodies can cause invading bacteria to dissolve, causing the inner substance of the bacteria to seep out into the body fluid, or they can combine with toxic antigens and thereby neutralize them.

When antibodies do their job, health is restored in the face of these hostile invading forces.

Natural immunity is a natural resistance against infections that you inherit genetically and with which you are born. Some people may have a high natural resistance to colds and flu, while others become ill every winter. However, a person's natural resistance to infectious diseases can be greatly enhanced or reduced by such factors as diet, environment, state of mental health, and the virulence of the currently circulating microorganisms.

Acquired immunity may either develop naturally within an individual's body, or develop artificially as a result of a vaccination or inoculation. When acquired immunity develops naturally, it results from a disease process within your body itself, and is produced during an initial attack by a causative bacterium or virus. When your body is invaded by a specific organism for the very first time, you may suffer a serious reaction. However, antibodies are built up against that initial invasion. A memory of the antigens produced is then passed on to successive generations of body cells. As a result, when your body is attacked again by the same antigen, the reaction might be very slight or there might be no reaction at all. Thus, you have acquired an immunity to an organism against which you had no natural immunity. This type of immunity, once developed, persists for years, or even for a lifetime. For example, smallpox confers lifelong immunity.

However, as every cold sufferer knows, colds

and many types of flu confer no immunity at all.

The Thymus Gland

Ancient philosophers considered the thymus gland to be the "seat of the soul," but modern immunologists regard the thymus as the "cornerstone of immunology." The thymus gland is important in immunology because the thymus acts as the site or origin for most of the antibody-forming cells that comprise the body's immune system.

Located in front of and above the heart, the cells of the thymus form rapidly during fetal and early life. This gland grows rapidly during the first two years of life and then atrophies during puberty. It is considered to be of vital importance during the early months of a child's life. It is responsible for the substances that serve to protect each one of us against invading bacteria and viruses. It is the birthplace of both lymphocytes (a variety of white blood cells responsible for defending our bodies—warrior immune cells), and plasma blood cells. Scientists have found that the thymus gland of an adult mouse can be removed with little effect, whereas a thymectomy in a newborn mouse results in either death or the failure of the mouse to respond to antigens with antibody formation, thus allowing the first invading bacteria or virus to take hold.

In the process of fighting off the invaders, a great variety of nutrients are required to forge the components of these cells, to sustain their efforts and to replenish their numbers and their efficiency when the battle against the invader is won.

Your body's resources for mounting and sustaining such an attack and the aftermath is not unlimited. A full complement of nutritional factors such as sleep, rest, proteins, vitamins, minerals and other substances is required for your body to emerge the winner in this constant battle.

Acid/Alkaline Balance

When your doctor takes a swab for a culture of your throat or nose in order to ascertain just what bacteria is growing there, he will send it out to a laboratory where it will be placed in a petri dish in a growth medium in order to be seen properly under a microscope.

Most infectious organisms have a preference for sweet and acid conditions in which to grow. Bacterial laboratories utilize growth media that contain sugar and that have an acid pH to prepare these cultures; they do that because this is the best "soil" for growing these micro-organisms.

The scientist's observation that most of these invaders prefer a sweet or acid environment suggests that a diet that is high in alkalinizing foods (most vegetables and fruits) and low in sugar will be beneficial to overall health, and will decrease the food for growth that these organisms rely on in the body.

When you have an active sinus infection, a diet low in sugar but high in nutrients should speed your recovery.

Colds and Flu

It is estimated that at any one time, over a third of the population has had a cold or the flu within the last two weeks. The national average is 2.5 colds per year—more than six hundred million colds in the US alone.

Colds and the flu are distinct and separate upper respiratory infections, triggered by different viruses. The flu is more serious than a cold, because it can spread to the lungs, causing severe bronchitis or pneumonia. In the beginning stages the symptoms for each condition may be very similar, because both colds and the flu begin when viruses penetrate the body's protective barriers.

The nose, eyes and the mouth are usually the sites of invasion for common cold viruses—such as the rhinovirus or the corona virus—and the most likely entry target for these viruses is the respiratory tract.

These viruses automatically activate an immune response. In order to control, ward off and defeat these invaders, the immune system must be in good health.

Drugs and over-the-counter medications only relieve the symptoms of these infections. They do not cure them, and often make the situation worse by depressing the immune response, drying up the mucous membranes and keeping the harmful invaders inside the body. Antibiotics are not effective against cold and flu viruses: they only go to work when there is an infection which *usually results* from the upper respiratory infection.

Therefore, it is important to keep the immune system healthy and strong.

The Common Cold

A cold has a slow onset and is rarely accompanied with fever and headache, often beginning with a sore throat You will have localized symptoms such as a runny nose and sneezing, with mild fatigue and some weakness. Sometimes there will be mild to moderate chest discomfort, occasionally accompanied by a dry cough.

It is best to get adequate rest, eat a nutritious diet, and maintain adequate hydration.

An analgesic such as acetaminophen will help decrease any muscle aches and pains.

With a healthy immune system, a cold will last approximately four days to a week.

The Flu

The flu—short for influenza—usually has a swift, severe onset with a feeling of fainting or weakness and flushed, hot, moist skin. There will be general symptoms of chills, depression and body aches. Sometimes there will be digestive symptoms of diarrhea and stomach ache. The sufferer often suffers extreme fatigue, which frequently lasts two to three weeks, accompanied by acute chest discomfort.

A fever is one of nature's methods for shortening the course of an infection—especially that of a virus—because heat interferes with the virus' ability to replicate itself.

If you are concerned about a child, it is OK for them to have a slight fever, *unless* you have an infant with a temperature over 100°F, or the fever has not abated after three days and is accompanied by vomiting, a cough and trouble breathing, or if the child is extremely lethargic and looks very ill. At that time the physician should be notified.

Bed rest during the acute stage of the illness and for 24 to 48 hours after the temperature becomes normal is recommended.

Adequate hydration and nutrition should be given.

Acetaminophen every four hours is helpful to ease the muscle discomfort that usually accompanies the illness.

A nasal decongestant can be given for temporary relief of symptoms.

Steam inhalation may relieve the respiratory symptoms and prevent drying of the nasal membranes.

Any complicating bacterial infections will require the attention of a physician and a course of appropriate antibiotics.

Section II

Sinusitis is the inflammation of the sinuses and can be caused by a number of factors.

When sinusitis occurs, mucus production *increases*, ciliary action to remove debris *decreases*, swelling of the mucous membranes *increases* and, infectious agents grow and multiply, trapped and incubated in this warm moist environment.

Mucus production can be triggered by an infectious agent (a virus or bacteria), a chemical pollutant, pollen, or other toxic agents in the environment. Any of them can stimulate the membrane lining of the sinuses to increase the production of mucus. This is initially a protective mechanism as the mucus is intended to enfold the foreign material and sweep it along for excretion.

When more mucus is being produced, the hairlike cilia cannot keep up with the amount being produced. They are engulfed in the mucus and can no longer perform their sweeping action to clean the sinus of debris at a rapid enough rate.

As a result, swelling of the mucous membrane begins to block the openings of the sinuses into the nasal cavity. These tiny ducts then an no longer drain, causing a back-up of mucus and other matter, increasing congestion and discomfort.

This swelling of the mucous membrane, and failure of the cilia to clear out debris, provides a moist, dark and warm environment, just right for bacteria or viruses to grow and multiply, creating a continuous condition of sinus injury.

The result: Sinusitis—headache and pain.

But, more than that, the sinuses are the body's leading barriers to injury or illness of the lungs, those essential vehicles for oxygen, vital to life itself. To stay healthy, we need to keep our sinuses well, for the well-being of the entire body.

Causes of Sinusitis

Viruses cause the common cold, and they are the most frequent cause of infections of the sinuses.

Next come the bacterias. Some of the common ones are *Streptococcus* (the bacteria which causes strep throat), *E. coli*, (the bacteria which is part of the normal flora of our intestines but can cause diarrhea or other illnesses if it finds its way to other body locations), and *Staphylococcus aureus*, (a bacteria which is commonly found on the skin).

A number of other conditions increase the chances of developing infected sinuses. The three most common conditions which predispose to sinusitis are: recurring colds, allergies, and excessive use of nose drops.

Additional things which increase the likelihood of sinus infections are: enlarged adenoids, nasal polyps, a deviated nasal septum, tumors, foreign bodies, swimming, diving, frequent flying, smoking or being exposed to secondary smoke.

If the sinus infection has been present for a short period, say no more than three weeks, it is considered acute. If longer, it is chronic. It is not unusual for sinusitis to remain for months, particularly if any of the additional things are present, such as frequent flying or allergies.

Acute sinusitis is typically diagnosed when there is pain or a feeling of pressure over the area of the infected sinuses. This pain can be made worse by bending over, straining, running or engaging in other strenuous activities. Pain or pressure may be accompanied by a cloudy nasal discharge or a postnasal drip and infrequently fever (which is not typical of chronic sinus conditions).

Chronic sinusitis is usually characterized by a constant nasal congestion or stuffiness, frequent recurring colds and a persistent cough.

In young children, it may seem as if the child always has a cold, has a nighttime cough and recurring ear infections.

For all sufferers, a cloudy postnasal drip, constant bad breath and recurring ear infections are common. Facial pain and fever usually do not accompany chronic sinusitis.

Rhinitis, the inflammation of the mucous membrane of the nose which usually accompanies a head cold, can become sinusitis which is chronic, particularly in those individuals who have: pain in the cheeks, at the base of the nose or around the eye sockets; a fever; pus coming out of the nose; a cold that won't get well or recurs frequently, or a cough that remains constant.

When anyone has frequent recurring symptoms or those symptoms are treated but the condition recurs, then chronic sinusitis should be considered.

Diagnosing Sinusitis

If symptoms appear to recur frequently, it is time to consider that the condition might be sinusitis, and it is wise to be examined by an otolaryngologist for a proper diagnosis, rather than just taking another course of antibiotics.

The otolaryngologist will examine the throat

and nose. With a special light, the doctor can examine the ducts that open into the nasal passageways. An X-ray of the sinuses may be necessary to identify swelling of the lining of the sinuses or the pooling of infected matter in any particular location.

Very infrequently, a CT (computerized tomographic X-ray) or a "CAT" scan is necessary. This is a more detailed examination of the sinuses and provides a better definition of the areas and of the extent of the condition.

Some conditions that may make one think they are suffering from sinusitis when one is not are:

Angioedema (allergic localized swelling)

This typically occurs on the face, around the nose or eyes and is due to localized swelling of the skin due to an allergic reaction. This swelling and tenderness near the eye socket can sometimes be mistaken for sinusitis.

Cellulitis

An infection of the skin and the tissues under the skin. The skin is red, warm to the touch and painful. If cellulitis occurs over the cheeks, at the base of the nose or around the eyes, it could be misdiagnosed as sinusitis.

Headache

Acute sinusitis is often accompanied with facial pain but most headaches can be helped with minor analgesia and are not connected to sinusitis.

Neuralgia of the trigeminal nerve

Intense pain shoots across the length of this nerve which is located in the face. This pain can be triggered by cold weather and is intense and sharp, differing from the dull pressure which accompanies sinusitis.

Temporal arteritis

Inflammation of a major artery which runs across the temple and usually involves only one side and is painful to the touch.

Toothache

Upper teeth are positioned quite near to the maxillary sinus cavities. In some individuals they actually touch the sinuses. The roots of the upper teeth and the maxillary sinuses are separated only by a paper-thin bone or sinus mucosa. Should any of these teeth become infected, that infection can irritate the lining of the sinuses and cause discomfort similar to sinusitis. An infection in a tooth can quickly extend into the sinus cavity and cause maxillary sinusitis. Toothache is a common symptom associated with an infection in these sinuses. Minor trauma, such as a tooth extraction, can easily perforate the sinus cavity—up to ten percent of maxillary sinus infections start with an infected tooth. Chewing or drinking hot beverages usually does not aggravate a sinus condition but will increase pain caused by an infected tooth.

Tumors

Many tumors of the nose do not produce symptoms until they have grown to a size sufficient to invade the surrounding tissue. When they do invade that tissue, pain ensues. However, such tumors are not usually accompanied by nasal drainage or that feeling of pressure which is typical of sinusitis.

The Goal of Treatment

If you have a head cold, your head is all stuffy and, after a week of feeling poorly and blowing your nose, it all clears up, fine.

But ...if you have repeated colds, are constantly stuffed up, unable to breathe freely, with draining in the back of the throat that wakes you up coughing in the middle of the night, it is time to do something about your sinuses. Untreated, a sinus infection can become a serious illness. A sinus filled with pus has the potential of becoming a brain abscess, meningitis, or an infection of the bone that surrounds the sinus, or of the skin and tissue around the eye. It can contribute to the development of chronic bronchial infections and can significantly aggravate bronchial asthma.

The goal of treatment of sinusitis includes:

promoting the drainage of the sinuses.

treating any infection.

avoiding the causes whenever possible.

Sometimes it takes some detective work to figure out just what those causes are: allergens, cigarette smoke, environmental pollution, dry air, cold air, dental conditions or malformations such as a deviated septum.

Tracking Down the Start of the Problem

If there were just one cause of sinus conditions, then being a detective and finding the cause, eliminating it from your life and getting your sinuses healthy would be quite easy. Unfortunately, that is seldom the case. Some factors may be more important than others: finding the cause of any illness is usually not that simple.

The Common Culprit

The beginning of sinus problems for most people is nothing more than the common cold, something almost everyone has experienced at some time or another. To never have a cold, you would have had to live in a plastic bubble in a laboratory in total isolation. The problem with that is that when you came out, you would be overwhelmed with diseases because your immune system would never have had the opportunity to develop any antibodies to anything in the outside world.

Colds are caused by viruses, something we are all exposed to on a daily basis. The main culprit in getting infected by the cold germs of others is our own hands. We touch things: the telephone, a pen, we shake hands with others, and then we, for a variety of reasons, touch our face, depositing the viruses there.

As the cold virus starts to grow inside the nose, the nasal mucous membrane becomes inflamed and swollen and the virus stops the cilia of the nasal membrane from doing their work of sweeping out debris. The result is that the mucus being produced by the sinuses cannot drain properly and this mucus becomes a breeding ground for more virus and bacteria, and then causes an infection.

Often after an individual has had one sinus infection, the mucous membrane and the cilia can be left damaged and weakened. For some, the membrane never completely recovers, especially in an environment that is not sinus-friendly. This assaulted and weakened sinus becomes more susceptible to additional infections from the next cold or other risk factors.

For someone who suffers from repeated sinus trouble, it is not enough to take a course of antibiotics, clear up the infection and then think the problem has been solved. This is the time to take a serious look at the complicating factors and attempt to remove them from your environment and your life.

Irritants

Smoke

After the common cold, cigarette smoking is probably number one in a list of possible culprits in continuous sinus problems.

Nicotine paralyzes the cilia. Super heated air also literally fries these hairlike projections. Once these tiny cilia have been stopped from their work of sweeping debris, that debris can move further down into the respiratory system, then germs can sit in the mucus, grow and multiply.

Cigarettes are not alone, however: cigars, pipes, campfires, cooking smoke can all cause damage, as well as other things that are smoked such as marijuana or cocaine. Cocaine snorted dries up the mucous membranes—that is just a part of its chemical makeup. Physicians who operate on nasal structures use a ten percent solution of cocaine to dry up the membrane to have a clear operating field, so its effect on this membrane is well documented.

Smoke of any kind irritates the mucous membrane. The greater the irritation, the more inflamed the membrane. An inflamed membrane swells and the more it swells, the more mucus it produces. Thus, the cycle continues: swelling, blocking the drainage ducts, causing more inflammation and then infection.

In 1992, a Harvard research team reported the first direct medical evidence that secondhand smoke can damage the lungs of nonsmokers. The study reported that secondhand smoke kills at least 4,000 people annually from lung cancer, increases the risk of respiratory infections in children and aggravates the symptoms of asthma in children.

Secondhand smoke can adversely affect the sinuses of those who already suffer from a sinus condition. Recent studies show that nonsmokers who live or work with smokers are also adversely affected. New laws that prohibit cigarette smoking in public places are definitely beneficial for those who need to avoid the smoke of others. The Cancer Society and the American Heart and Lung Association cite thousands of documents that substantiate the adverse effects of cigarette smoking on the health of the American public. The passage of laws on the state level which limit the smoking permitted in public places indicates thinking on the part of lawmakers that the rights of nonsmokers should take precedence over the rights of smokers, when both are in public environments.

When antismoking legislation began, many smokers opposed such laws, stating it was within their rights as Americans to continue to smoke. The militant anti-smokers had a slogan which was, "Your right to smoke ends at my nose." State legislators apparently recognized that it is not possible for the smoker to contain the smoke from his or her tobacco product and legislation passed which prohibits smoking in public places stated that smokers were, in effect, invading the rights of others.

The American Heart Association has estimated that, in addition to its adverse effects on lungs, secondhand smoke could be a contributing factor in the heart disease deaths of forty thousand non-smoking Americans every year. They estimate that fifty million nonsmoking adults over the age of thirty-five are exposed to secondhand smoke and about fifty percent of all American children live in families with one or more smokers.

Because the sinuses and their condition seem secondary to the effects of smoke on the lungs and hearts, not much attention has been paid to them in these studies. However it is obvious that when such statistical evidence points to the damage that smoke does to those structures, secondhand smoke obviously must also causes significant damage to the first line of defense of the heart and lungs: the body's air filtering system.

Air Pollution—Outdoor

The word "smog" is a fairly recent one in the vocabulary of most Americans. You might have to look in a dictionary of slang to find a definition. However, everyone knows what it is and everyone has seen it. It is a visible brownish haze in the sky above many cities. Now most cities of the world are frequently covered by this thick layer of dirty air, particularly those situated in valleys.

Hawaii, once known for its clear air that was swept clean by the trade winds, has a serious smog problem. The great increase in the number of automobiles pumping out tons of exhaust daily, the building of high-rise hotels along the beaches, have contributed to the problem by trapping the auto exhaust and other air pollutants inside the ring of these high-rise buildings. Where the trade winds once blew across these islands freely, industrialization has created a problem for hundreds of thousands of residents and visitors.

This kind of a smog-filled air problem is present in almost all industrialized regions of the world. Mexico City and Cairo, Egypt, for example, now have such air pollution that many people can no longer live there. In some areas where temperature inversions are frequent—warm air up higher trapping cold air and the pollutants below it—smog-alerts or air pollution alerts must be broadcast daily, so that those with breathing problems or other respiratory difficulties can plan to remain indoors.

Scientific evidence points to carbon monoxide as the most dangerous element in air pollution and about twenty-five percent of that is from motor vehicles. In sufficient concentrations, carbon monoxide can kill. It is also one of the components of air pollution measured by the Environmental Protection Agency (EPA). Their standard for small particulates—less than ten microns in diameter— is considered hazardous when the ambient air contains 150 microns of these particles per cubic meter. It takes far less than this to make people sick. The larger particulates—more than ten microns in diameter—are not measured by the EPA. The EPA prepares an annual report on national air quality (referring only to those smaller PM-10 particulates and emissions) and it lists the metropolitan areas with the highest eight-hour concentrations of carbon monoxide in the previous year.

Carbon monoxide, which makes up twenty-five percent of smog, is a colorless, odorless gas. The other seventy-five percent that makes up the visible components of smog, the stuff that makes it hang over our heads in a brown ugly cloud, consists of oxides of sulfur, oxides of nitrogen, hydrocarbons and ozone, plus tiny particles of dust, sand, cinders, soot, smoke.

Where does it all come from? Carbon monoxide comes chiefly from the exhaust of motor vehicles of all types: cars, buses, trucks, farm machinery, power boats. The rest comes from roads, fields, construction, factories, power plants, burning of rubbish, wood-burning stoves, dust and pollen.

When we breathe, we inhale the ambient air of our environment, whether it is polluted or not. We have no choice, breathing is absolutely essential to human life. Sometimes the pollution in the air is visible, as everyone knows who has ever sat in a traffic jam behind a big diesel truck. It doesn't take much to realize that the dark cloud coming out of the truck's exhaust isn't good for us. The awful smell of those fumes often is enough to make most people nauseated after breathing them in for only a few minutes.

Larger particles (10 microns or more in diameter) are often trapped in the nose and sinuses. Trapping these foreign particles is one of the main functions of those structures, protecting the respiratory system from damage. Smaller particles (less than 10 microns), can get past this filtering system. These very tiny particulates do the most damage to the sinuses and the other structures of the respiratory system, including the lungs.

Unfortunately, the Environmental Protection Agency's standard for airborne particulates measuring 10 microns or smaller is still not sufficient to protect children's health. Environmental economist Arden Pope III of Brigham Young University in Provo, Utah, found that bronchitis and asthma hospitalizations for children living near a sub-10-emitting steel plant were lower when the plant closed for thirteen months and again higher when the plant reopened.

Douglas Dockery of the Harvard School of Public Health in Boston reported that children living in cities with high levels of airborne particulates measuring 15 microns or less had a much greater bronchitis risk than children living in cities with low particulate levels.

Studies reported by the Environmental Protection Agency estimate that as many as sixty thousand people die each year as the result of inhaling particulate pollution. The most harmful particles are those less than 10 microns in size and these are produced chiefly by industrial plants and the exhaust of diesel vehicles.

The United States alone spends about $35 billion a year on scrubbers, catalytic converters, and other air pollution control devices with only one-third of that funding aimed at particulates. Of that one-third, only a fraction is aimed at the smaller particles. Most regulatory efforts have focused on pollutants which have been well documented to adversely damage the health of the population, such as sulfur dioxide.

Sulfur dioxide is emitted mainly by coal and oil-powered power plants, refineries and pulp and paper mills. It is well documented that oxides of sulfur are irritating to the bronchial mucosa, damage the cilia and contribute to bronchitis.

Nitrogen oxides form when fuel is burned at high temperatures. Major sources of these emissions are motor vehicles, aircraft, and electric utilities. When produced, these oxides contribute the ugly yellowish-brown color to smog. Just as sulfur irritates the mucosa, nitrogen oxides irritate the lungs, cause bronchitis and contribute to pneumonia. It is also thought that these particulates impair the body's immune system, making an individual more susceptible to bacterial and viral infections.

Hydrocarbons have been well documented to be highly irritating to the mucous membranes of the body. Hydrocarbons are evaporated or incompletely burned organic compounds. The largest sources of hydrocarbons include internal combustion engines, certain industrial processes, such as coke ovens in steel mills, and the evaporation of liquids, such as gasoline and industrial and household solvents. Legislation has recently been passed that requires gas stations to make a closer seal around the gas pump and the gas tank of motor vehicles to prevent the evaporation of these fuels during fueling.

Ozone is produced when sunlight acts on nitrogen oxide and hydrocarbons. Ozone in the breathable part of the atmosphere (within 1,000 feet of the earth's surface) is harmful to human and animal health, crops, and forests. Ozone can cause shortness of breath and coughing during exercise in healthy adults and it has more serious effects on the health of both the young and the elderly. It is known to adversely affect the respiratory system. Ozone in the upper atmosphere is beneficial as it absorbs the harmful rays of sunlight. Legislation has been passed in the United States preventing the use of aerosol sprays that use fluorocarbons as a propellant, in air conditioning and refrigerators. However, many other nations continue to allow their use, causing the depletion of the ozone layer in the upper atmosphere and possibly contributing to global warming and to other health hazards related to ultraviolet rays from the sun.

Acid rain, the result of these particles falling back to earth, has been a serious cause of conflict between the U.S. and Canada in recent years because the emissions of industrial plants are being considered the cause of the destruction of large tracts of forest. The problem of acid rain has caused a serious destruction of forests all across central Europe. When these particles fall back to earth they further compound the hazard of ozone for humans and animals in the breathable part of the earth's atmosphere.

The World Health Organization states that asthma, emphysema, chronic bronchitis and lung cancer have increased by fifty percent since 1981. The American Lung Association estimates that the annual costs associated with pollution-related illnesses range from $40 billion to $50 billion.

Each of us need to take steps to encourage a reduction in environmental pollution. We can support legislation that forces industry to clean up its factories and plants, encourage the development of solar energy, and the use of alternative fuels.

Motor vehicles are the main sources of air pollution. Therefore, individually each of us can actively be a part of the solution rather than the problem. We can cooperate with emission tests on our automobiles, maintain our vehicles properly, and be thoughtful about acts which might, even in a small way, add to the outdoor pollution.

Air Pollution—Indoor

Americans spend approximately ninety percent of their time indoors. We are either at home, at work, or in large indoor spaces such as the mall, grocery stores, theaters or sports arenas. More people work in offices than work outdoors, and those people go from the home to the car to the office, back into the car and home again, for a majority of their waking hours. Unfortunately, staying inside does not protect anyone against air pollution.

The World Health Organization estimates that thirty percent of new or remodeled commercial buildings generate an unusual number of health and illness complaints. Nearly one fifth of the work force in the United States has reported indoor air pollution ailments which range from headaches and fatigue to colds, influenza and chronic respiratory illness. One million hospital visits per year are attributed to poor indoor air quality alone.

Pollutants

Fumes from motor vehicles

Sources include outdoor traffic, outdoor parking lots, indoor garages, gas stations.

Chemicals

Sources include interior artifacts—formaldehyde used in insulation, fiberboard, furniture. Petroleum based chemicals used in the manufacture of furniture and carpeting. Cleaning solutions—carpet cleaning solutions, oven cleaners, etc. Solvents in paints and dry cleaning materials; aerosol sprays. Chemicals used in the maintenance of indoor equipment such as copiers, computers, etc.

Particulates

These include dust, pollen, animal dander and asbestos.

Smoke from combustion

Household smoke (tobacco, wood burning fireplaces, stoves).

Fuel from gas operated appliances (clothes dryers, water heaters, stoves).

Microorganisms

Microorganisms inclue bacteria, viruses, molds, fungi and dust mites.

Humidifiers, air conditioners, or other damp conditions allow these microorganisms to grow.

Sick Building Syndrome is thought to result from microorganisms which have flourished in air conditioning systems and then been pumped through the air, invading offices and making large numbers of workers ill with respiratory disease.

Radio nuclides

Radon—a radioactive gas that is emitted from the earth and enters through basements, crawl spaces and the water supply. This gas attaches itself to the particulates of cigarette smoke, dust particles and aerosols.

Ion imbalance

Excessive positive ions

Energy efficient buildings have constantly re-circulated air which leads to a depletion of the beneficial negative ions and a subsequent increase in positive ions. It has been found that areas of low negative ions or an excess of positive ions contribute to feelings of ill health.

Tightly sealed homes designed for lowered energy costs and energy-efficient living may not be the best idea because this creates a condition of low ventilation. High rise buildings and the current trend to provide glass that office workers can look through but cannot open has replaced natural ventilation with artificial ventilation by energy efficient heating and air conditioning. Without any type of natural air exchange, pollutants can be trapped inside office buildings and homes, resulting in sick air for the inhabitants to breathe.

The Effects of Cold Air

Everyone who has experienced very cold weather knows that one of the first things that happens with such exposure is a runny nose. One of the tasks of both the nose and the sinuses is to warm the incoming air before it goes to the lungs. This runny nose in cold weather occurs as a result of inhaling cold air—not because you have a cold or a sinus condition. When it is hit by extremely cold air, the mucous membrane begins to defend against this onslaught of cold air by mucous production and the result is a runny nose.

Studies have recently shown that healthy individuals who exercise or perform other physical activities such as running, skating or skiing in extremely cold weather, or those whose work keeps them outdoors in very cold weather, can develop adult-onset asthma.

For anyone with a chronic sinus condition, the air-warming functions of the nose and sinuses may already be impaired. Cold air is often more humid, but the shock of the temperature to the mucous membrane can create irritation and injury to those all-important tiny hairlike cilia.

The Effects of Dry Air

We already know that one of the important functions of the sinuses is to humidify incoming air.

Dry air can be another climate that makes it difficult for the proper functioning of the sinuses. As a response to the lack of moisture, they may work excessively to produce the proper moisture, making the secretory cells of the internal nose work overtime in an attempt to humidity the incoming air, and the cilia then will have to struggle to keep the mucus that is produced moving.

At one time there was a television commercial that showed a man suffering with a sinus condition. His sinuses took wing and then flew away to a dry climate while he breathed a sigh of relief. Unfortunately, this was merely a commercial, an attempt to stimulate sales of a product that dried up a runny nose or attempted to control postnasal drip; it was not reality.

As we have already seen, a dry climate is not the answer. In fact, individuals who live in arid climates may find that their sinus condition is worse rather than better. The same is true of high elevations, such as at ski resorts, because the higher the elevation, the dryer the air.

To understand this concept, think of the effect of forced-air heating systems when you wake up with an uncomfortable dry throat and a drier nose. You are not cold, you are not exposed to the shock of cold, damp air, but the condition of your sinuses tells you that dry air has not been beneficial. Sometimes older heating systems make it necessary to add moisturizing drops to the nose in order to feel comfortable again. Air conditioning too, can have a drying effect.

Many older heating systems and air conditioners do not have a way to either moisturize or dry the air. However it may be possible to add such a unit in order to maintain the moisture content at forty to sixty percent humidity, the right humidity for proper functioning of the mucous membrane. Too much moisture can create an environment where many microorganisms, such as bacteria, viruses, molds and fungi can grow, particularly if the humidity exceeds sixty percent.

If you have sinusitis, you should examine both the heating and air-conditioning systems in your home to be sure they provide the proper moisture balance for a healthy respiratory system.

Allergy

An allergy attack is actually a defensive and protective response. It is an attempt by the body to neutralize and destroy agents the body views as toxic or a threat before they can travel further into the body. The allergen stimulates the mucous membrane of the nose to release a chemical called histamine. *Histamine* is believed to increase the diameter of the blood vessels, or dilate them. It also increases the permeability of the plasma membranes of the blood vessel cells. Dilation increases the amount of blood that can enter the area. And the increase in permeability allows defensive substances in the blood to pass through the vessel walls and into the injured tissue. Such defensive substances include white blood cells, antibodies, oxygen and other chemicals. The increased blood supply also carries off poisonous products and dead cells, preventing them from complicating the insult to the tissue.

The body responds further by increasing its metabolic rate and insuring that more blood circulates to the area. This large increase in histamine and other defensive substances causes tissue inflammation and the contraction of smooth muscle fibers. When this occurs in the breathing tubes and the blood vessels, it causes them to constrict.

Such an allergic reaction causes the mucous membrane to swell with resultant blockage of the sinus ducts, reduced action of the cilia and then filled sinuses. Sneezing (the body's effort to remove the offending allergen), the runny nose, the moist eyes, are more than annoying. If allowed to continue, they are all part of creating a climate just right for the development of a sinus infection.

Most people are unaware of just what it is they are allergic to. It could be any of thousands of things: grass, weeds, flowers, mold, animals. Sometimes people who have been tested and find they are allergic to something in particular think they should move away from the thing that causes their allergic reaction and discomfort. However, allergic individuals usually find that moving does not solve the problem. After a while of being away from the offending substance, they find that they are now allergic again—to something new. The reason for this is that repeated exposure to the new substance causes the immune response to it that results in the allergic symptoms.

Food Allergies

Frequently food allergies cause allergic symptoms less than an hour after eating, and may affect only limited areas of the body—the skin, the airways, and the digestive tract.

Many experts have dismissed food allergy as a serious threat, especially to adults. Even among children, they claim, only ten percent are affected by food allergy, and that, they suggest, is often quickly outgrown. Adult food allergies are often not taken seriously unless they conform to the same symptomatic patterns seen in the immediate allergic responses: stuffy nose, wheezing, hives, or gastrointestinal upset occurring shortly after eating the allergenic food.

Food allergy is by definition an irritation of tissues, or inflammation, caused by a food allergen. Where an allergen decides to deposit itself and do its damage is probably predetermined genetically. Everyone has physiological and biochemical strong and weak points—diseases they are resistant to and those they are susceptible to.

Ten people allergic to milk may react to it in ten highly individual ways. It might cause migraine headaches in one, diarrhea in another, a flare-up of rheumatoid arthritis in another. More and more frequently, those with sinusitis are considering that food allergy might be at the root of their problem. Symptoms are usually not sudden reactions but have built up over time. In fact, one of the insidious aspects of most food allergy reactions is that the majority of symptoms, at least in the early developmental stages, are mild and seem to have no direct connection to the food.

Some symptoms are especially frequent indicators of food allergy. One is fatigue. Though many disease states may be associated with chronic fatigue, perhaps the most common cause is food and chemical hypersensitivity, particularly if the tired feeling shows up after meals, or upon awakening in the morning, or is associated with other symptoms of allergy, such as sinusitis.

Allergic shiners (dark circles under the eyes), swelling or puffiness under the eyes or wrinkles under the eyes are frequently traceable to allergy. One other very common symptom, familiar to all those with sinusitis, is excess mucus formation— characterized by a chronically congested nose, postnasal drip and excessive phlegm.

Most methods of self-testing for food allergy can be difficult and time-consuming, but they can pinpoint your allergies with a reasonable degree of accuracy if carefully monitored. Also, if you suspect a food allergy, you might want to try self-testing for screening purposes before going ahead with any further expensive clinical testing.

If you have very obvious symptoms, such as migraine headaches, a chronic runny or stuffy nose, fatigue or insomnia, you already have a barometer by which to measure your responses.

Allergic reactions to food are the result not only of eating the allergenic food, but of the amount eaten, your general health at the time, and cumulative stress, as well as other foods or beverages eaten in combination with the suspect food. This begins to look like a complex equation but with a little effort, it can be simplified.

It is difficult to test food allergies accurately if you are taking medications, especially the ones most frequently used by people with allergies and inflammatory disease such as antihistamines or anti-inflammatories. To test for food allergy, you should ask your physician if it will be OK to temporarily stop your medications.

When allergens are thought to be caused by food, physicians usually have the patient try an elimination diet. To do this, you eliminate from your diet any foods you suspect to be allergens for a full five days and then reintroduce each food one at a time to see whether it provokes an allergic response.

It is difficult to test every food you eat to see if you are allergic, but here are some guidelines if you decide you want to try an elimination diet.

List the foods you know you have some kind of a reaction to (foods that frequently disagree with you—cause your nose to run, or your eyes to water, not just stomach upsets) and the foods you eat most often and probably prefer. This frequent list should include foods that you eat every three days or so, or even more frequently. This might include coffee, flavorings, and all the ingredients in processed foods that you eat frequently. One of the problems with having a favorite food, e.g. chocolate or ice cream, is that overloading on one particular food means that you place an extreme burden on the immune response if that particular food turns out to be the allergen to which you are having your reaction.

Abstain from five foods on this list for a full five days; the five foods you suspect the most. It is important to read labels carefully on any packaged foods during this period—eggs, wheat, sugar and corn, for example, show up in a great variety of foods. The easiest way to avoid hidden ingredients is to eat simple, fresh whole foods. With some thought you can devise a diet that avoids all the suspected foods and eat only infrequently consumed foods for these five days. Then carefully reintroduce the suspected allergenic foods one at a time and note your reaction. Five days is necessary because it takes that long for most allergic symptoms to be removed so that reintroducing the food might provoke a reaction.

The reintroduction process is as follows:

After five days, take your resting pulse and then eat a substantial, unseasoned portion of the suspect food, by itself, as the first food of the day.

While resting in unstressful surroundings, take your pulse again fifteen minutes later, and every fifteen minutes for the next hour and a half. If your pulse increases b twelve to sixteen beats, unexplained by stress or activity, you should suspect a food allergy. In addition, monitor your other symptoms, particularly those you have experienced before. Look for feelings of body heat, itching, a stuffy nose, a headache. If you experience strong symptoms, you should suspect food allergy. Let six hours lapse before eating your next meal. The majority of delayed symptoms will appear within one to six hours after eating. Remember that many allergic reactions will not appear right away.

Test each food on your list, one at a time, using this method each day.

Because you are not eating the foods you suspect cause your allergies, you might find that you feel uncomfortable or have detoxification symptoms for the first few days, but it should not be difficult to distinguish these from allergic reactions. You might feel shaky or have a frontal headache, symptoms which are often related to changes in blood sugar levels and different from allergic symptoms.

While this might seem to be a complicated process, it is what the physician who suspects a food allergy will ask you to do in order to evaluate your allergic reaction to foods. An elimination diet is much simpler than eliminating allergens which are airborne, because the item of food can be controlled. An elimination diet can often pinpoint particular foods such as wheat, dairy products, artificial food coloring, or eggs, for example. When the substance is identified, it is often possible to add it back into the diet in very slow increments, without creating any difficulty. What this pinpoints is a concept that is fairly easy to understand, that the body has a tolerance level, after which it creates an allergic reaction in order to protect against the offending substance.

If you find foods are causing allergic reactions and contributing to your sinusitis, it may be possible to eliminate those foods either by substituting others that contribute the same elements to your diet, or eliminating them altogether (such as chocolate or caffeine), and you should soon begin to feel healthier—which can be well worth the trouble and time a brief elimination diet takes.

Air Borne Allergens

In the case of airborne allergens it may be easy to eliminate some of them (pet dander, for example) but it is very difficult to control the air we breathe and the substances that are floating around in it. However efforts to reduce allergens, particularly in the bedroom (where we spend a third of our time) can make a substantial difference.

Those with allergies are very susceptible to sinusitis because of the continuous hyperactive and hyper-secretory activity of the nasal and sinus mucosae. If allergies are a year-round problem, chronic sinusitis should also be considered.

Hazardous Occupations

Exposure to conditions of adverse air can be an obvious contributor to chronic sinusitis. Some of the occupations considered high risk for this condition are obvious, such as fire fighters, auto mechanics, taxi drivers, painters, farmers, and parking garage attendants. Others who are at risk that might not be as immediately obvious are airline personnel, police officers and beauticians.

Anyone who suffers from a sinus condition should consider the ventilation of the work place before accepting employment. If there are choices, make them for your own health.

Anyone with a chronic sinus condition should consider the exposure to toxic air of any occupation before undertaking it, where at all possible.

If it is not possible to change occupations,

take steps to control your personal environment, such as asking questions about the filtering system on the air conditioning system in your work place. This can be done without creating difficulties: volunteer to be on a safety committee, for example. Remember, you are helping protect the air your employer breathes too.

Contributing Physical Factors

The most common contributory physical factor to developing sinusitis is a deviated septum. The septum is the wall that separates the two sides of the nose. It is not unusual for this structure to be more to one side or the other. In some cases, one side of the nose is entirely blocked off by this septum, making breathing out of that side of the nose difficult or impossible.

Most deviated septa are present from birth and can be repaired surgically.

Other things that can cause obstruction of the ostia, the ducts that drain the sinuses, are enlarged adenoids, cysts or polyps. All can be diagnosed readily and corrected by an otolaryngologist.

Adenoids

This tissue normally exists in the nasopharynx of children and is known as the pharyngeal tonsil. This tissue can become enlarged or overgrown.

Cyst

A cyst is a small sac that may contain liquid or a semisolid substance. Cysts sometimes occur around a foreign body or as a result of overgrowth of the mucous membrane.

Polyp

This is a growth on a short stem that arises from the mucosa and extends into the nose as a result of the overgrowth of the mucous membrane.

Symptoms of Sinusitis

It would seem that diagnosing sinusitis would be simple. You have pain or pressure right above your eyes and you can't breathe because of a stuffy nose. Should be relatively simple, even your Aunt Martha can tell you what is wrong. The problem is most sinus conditions start as nothing more than a common cold. Usually after a week or more, the cold symptoms improve and most of us forget the cold until we get another.

When a sinus condition becomes chronic, you will find that the simple common cold is much worse, or was gone for a couple of weeks and now you think you have another cold. You might complain, "I've just had one cold after another this year, guess it must be the cold weather or it must be the damp weather, or those kids brought home some new germs from school this year," or some other reason with which you attempt to explain why this cold hangs on and on.

When it finally becomes worrisome enough to call for an appointment with the doctor, frequently as much as a year has gone by. A common complaint is that you haven't felt well all this year. You've had frequent colds or the cold that you got last fall never really went away. Often it is only when the symptoms are acute, such as pain or fever, that many people will take their sinus condition to a physician for diagnosis.

A CT scan (computerized tomographic X-ray) or "CAT" scan is the ultimate diagnostic tool for sinusitis. Almost ninety percent of individuals who thought they just had a "summer cold" or a "cold I can't shake" actually were suffering from an infected sinus, as diagnosed by a CAT scan. Unfortunately, a CAT scan is both costly and inconvenient.

Colds

A common cold is a viral infection of the nasal and often sinus mucous membranes, usually preceded by a sore throat. The symptoms are a stuffy and runny nose with a thin clear or white mucus, fatigue, and mild muscle aches. Additional symptoms might include a headache, persistent sore throat, cough, and a low-grade fever. The average cold lasts approximately four to seven days. If the cough persists and the fever increases, the sufferer now has something else, possibly bronchitis.

Bronchitis

Bronchitis is part of an upper respiratory tract infection. It may develop following the common cold or other viral infection of the nasopharynx, throat or the tracheobronchial tree, often with a secondary bacterial infection. Exposure to air pollutants, and possibly chilling and fatigue, can contribute to bronchitis.

It is possible to have both bronchitis and sinusitis. They have a common origin—the common cold. The symptoms are similar. They are those of an acute upper respiratory infection: fatigue, slight fever, back and muscle pain, and a sore throat.

What differentiates bronchitis from sinusitis is the onset of a cough. The cough is initially dry and nonproductive, but small amounts of sputum can be raised after only a few hours. This sputum may become more abundant as the disease progresses. A fever to 101-102°F may be present for as long as a week; then acute symptoms usually subside, although the cough may continue for several weeks. Persistent fever for longer than this suggests a complicating pneumonia.

Sinusitis

If the sinuses have been weakened by prior infections, the common cold can quickly cause renewed problems. Within the first few days of a cold, symptoms of a sinus infection might occur. These symptoms, the speed with which they appear and the severity of them, are determined by the already existing condition of the sinus tissue.

The most common symptoms that cause someone to seek medical attention for a sinus infection are the cough and the sore throat that cause the most discomfort, and keep one from sleeping.

Cough

A cough can be diagnosed as caused by a number of other conditions, including bronchitis. The damp, mucus cough of bronchitis is felt deep in the chest, as opposed to the dry tickling kind of cough from the throat that is typical of sinusitis.

The cough of a sinus infection worsens when you lie down at night. The cough of bronchitis is persistent throughout the day.

Adults' postnasal drip goes down the back of the throat during the daytime, keeping it away from the trachea and into the stomach. Sometimes, if the sufferer has had the condition for a long time, this swallowing of the mucus from a postnasal drip becomes almost an unconscious behavior.

Head congestion

Head congestion is most obvious early in the morning. There may be a feeling of fullness in the head, as well in the nose. A hot shower may bring some relief.

Senses of smell and taste

The voice may be altered, the senses of smell and taste may be diminished.

Dull ache

There can be a dull ache behind the eyes.

Dizziness

Sometimes dizziness and a feeling of being light-headed are present.

Headache

Headache may or not be present, but when one is, it often pinpoints the location of the affected sinus. Sinus headaches tend to worsen when you bend forward or lie down and are most often worse in the morning and ease later in the day.

Facial pain

In acute sinusitis, there may be pain as well as swelling in the region of the infected sinus. This is caused by the air, pus and mucus being trapped within that body.

An infected maxillary sinus will cause pain and sometimes swelling in the area over the affected sinus, at the cheek. Pain may occur under the eye or in the upper teeth, particularly the molars. When air is prevented from entering the sinus by the swollen mucous membrane, a vacuum can be created, resulting in severe pain. When the barometric pressure drops because of weather changes or during the landing of an airplane, when the pressure in the airplane cabin is lowered, the pressure on the duct draining the sinus is increased.

An infected ethmoid sinus produces pain between and behind the eyes, and tenderness when pressure is applied to the sides of the nose.

An infected frontal sinus causes pain in the forehead and over the eyes.

An infected sphenoid sinus produces a generalized pain, deep in the head, usually at the back of the head near the base of the skull, which becomes aggravated whenever the head is moved rapidly. The infection of this sinus usually creates the symptom of dizziness or light-headedness.

Children often experience facial pain accompanied by swelling of the orbit of the eye that involves the upper eyelid. The swelling is most obvious in the morning, upon arising. Children also experience photo phobia, an unwillingness to open the eyes in bright light.

Fatigue

Fatigue can sometimes be the chief complaint. Since chronic sinusitis is a systemic illness, an infection that is not getting better or worse, it actually affects the entire body. Fatigue can be accompanied by irritability. You are sleeping more at night, having difficulty surviving a full day at work, taking naps. For those individuals who are accustomed to exercising regularly, there is a drop-off in the desire to continue your workouts because of extreme fatigue. Once you begin excusing yourself because of tiredness, it is very easy to find a reason to discontinue all exercise until you feel better, whenever that might be.

When this condition continues for weeks and sometimes months, it is easy to become accustomed to this level of general malaise or discomfort. You may have difficulty recalling the last time you really felt well.

Fatigue is a condition that is common to many other ailments, and if this is the only complaint, other diagnoses might be given before the sinuses are found to be the cause. Misdiagnosis is common because the precipitating factor might be a common cold you suffered last year, or months ago and have already forgotten.

Mucus production

Yellow-green mucus is a classic symptom of sinusitis in children. Most of us have seen children
with a runny nose wiping such mucus on the back
of a sleeve and looked away in disgust. However,
the child is suffering from an infection which needs
to be treated.

The mucus in adults, however, is often not
yellow at all. It may be yellow, clear, or white, or
there may be no mucus from the nose at all. In
adult sinusitis the mucus may be draining down
the back of the throat. Many adults are unaware
of this constant drip down the back of the throat,
they have become so accustomed to its presence.

However, if you have to cough up mucus or
are aware of it first thing in the morning, and find
that it diminishes during the day, you might very
well have an infected sinus.

If you suspect your sinuses are infected, spit
into a tissue first thing in the morning, examine
the mucus you have produced during the night
and you could be able to make your own correct
diagnosis immediately. This is one of the few objective signs of acute sinusitis and it is consistently present.

Nasal Congestion

A stuffy and runny nose is one of the primary symptoms of the common cold. A cold almost always precedes a sinus infection. Sometimes the sinus infection follows the cold closely.

In adults, stuffy nose is more prevalent than runny nose and often present on only one side.

In children, the yellow nasal discharge can be copious.

Fever

Fever will usually appear early in the course of any infection, before other symptoms are obvious. However, fevers accompany many different infections.

Hoarseness

Hoarseness or laryngitis results from many of the same factors that cause the throat to be sore and irritated. Postnasal mucus draining down into the larynx causes irritation and inflammation of the vocal cords and the cartilage in the larynx.

Irritated throat

Postnasal drip down the back of the throat can irritate the throat.

Mouth breathing, particularly at night because of congestion in the nose, can cause a sore, dry throat which is usually worse upon awakening than it is later in the day.

Lack of humidity can also contribute to a sore throat, particularly if you cannot breathe through the nose, or sleep with your mouth open in order to breathe in a poorly humidified room.

Unfortunately, the clinical picture of acute sinusitis varies greatly: some people are quite sick, while others are only minimally uncomfortable.

In an adult, a common cold followed by head congestion, headache, extreme fatigue and post-nasal drip are the usual symptoms of sinusitis.

In a child, yellow-green nasal mucus—usually from one nostril—a fever, foul-smelling breath, and a cough are the usual symptoms of sinusitis.

Duration

Five to seven days.

Diagnosing Chronic Sinusitis

The National Center for Health Statistics states chronic sinusitis is the most common chronic disease in the United States. It is more common in women, reaching a peak among women between ages forty-five to sixty-five. Twenty-two percent of all women in this age category have the condition as compared to fifteen percent of men.

Rhinitis is an irritation of the lining of the nose, and sinusitis is a complication of rhinitis.

That irritation can be caused by an allergen, a chemical, an irritation or an infection, but usually is caused by the common cold virus. Sinusitis is a medical term that means any inflammation of the sinuses, and that inflammation can be caused by a variety of factors. Usually it is caused by an infection—most likely by the common cold virus with all its usual symptoms that usually last from five to seven days.

Many people suffer from a chronic sinus condition for years without really being aware of it. You might have nasal congestion, a runny nose or postnasal drip, a poor sense of smell or a diminished sense of taste. Because you have lived with this condition for years, you may have just accepted it as being normal for you. Because you are not experiencing the symptoms that usually take people to the doctor (the headache, the fever, the aching teeth) you may be unaware that you have a sinus condition. You may have accepted this condition as "just the way things are."

You might find that you are more sensitive to cigarette smoke, dry air, cold air, or certain other pollution, such as exhaust fumes. Many people experience this kind of increased sensitivity but say nothing about it, not wanting to be considered an antismoking nut or a chronic complainer. Or you might casually remark, "Guess my allergies are in full bloom today," or "Cigarette smoke always makes my eyes water."

Many people don't realize just what is happening to the mucous membranes as the result of exposure to these irritants, don't realize that it isn't allergy, it isn't a sensitive nose, it isn't some bizarre fixation on a particular odor; it is a chronic sinus condition.

The longer you are exposed to any of these irritants, the more likely you will be to develop a sinus infection. This is because there is a chronic inflammation of the mucous membrane of the nose and sinuses as the result of the irritants—possibly with an infrequent infection or no infection at all. The continual exposure to these irritants has caused swelling and increased secretions from the mucous membranes but these membranes have not become the dwelling sites of any of the infectious agents, such as the viruses or fungi—yet.

As time goes by, there is a gradual weakening of the mucous membrane due to the chronic inflammation, a decrease in the natural resistance to infection because a normal, not swollen, mucosa is able to protect against infection, while a chronically inflamed membrane cannot.

An ordinary, run-of-the-mill cold, which should last about a week, can turn into a sinus infection, and then the colds become more and more frequent. This cycle continues with weaker and weaker sinus membranes, resulting in more infections. Finally, the simple common cold is a frequent visitor because however it begins, whether it starts out as "just a cold" that turns into bronchitis, a bout with the flu that leaves you weak and debilitated, an allergy attack that tires you out with the sneezing and the headache, they all end up in the sinuses as a sinus infection. Your sinuses, weak and damaged, have become your Achilles heel, the weakest, most vulnerable part of your body.

Acute Sinusitis

Usually preceded by a common cold with all the usual symptoms: a sore throat, cough, hoarseness, headache, nasal congestion with thin, clear nasal mucus, fatigue, muscle ache, headache, and a low-grade fever.

Often preceded by allergies or exposure to pollutants (such as cigarette smoke).

Now the symptoms may include facial pain and headache, thick yellow nasal mucus, postnasal drainage (often draining down the back of the throat during sleep) and extreme fatigue.

And these symptoms last beyond the usual

week to ten days of the common cold.

Acute sinusitis is caused by a variety of pathogens and usually begins with a viral respiratory tract infection—or the common cold. Recurring acute infections can appear to happen almost simultaneously with the onset of the cold and recur frequently. All the symptoms are there and the sufferer will frequently say, "As soon as I get a cold, it goes right to my sinuses." What might have started out as "just a cold" becomes an immediate sinus infection in the weakened and damaged mucous membranes.

Even after treatment with antibiotics, you may consider yourself cured when the headache and fever are gone, but you will continue to live with a stuffy nose, a lower-level headache and chronic postnasal drip. This scenario may be repeated frequently during the year, with the "summer cold," the "winter cold," the "spring allergy attack," and the "fall leaves stuffy nose syndrome."

Perhaps it is allergy or just another cold, but it is usually the damaged and weakened sinus and nasal mucous membrane, repeatedly assaulted and becoming a breeding ground for bacteria, that results in frequent sinus infections. These infections may require a treatment with antibiotics to clear them up, until the next one. This is acute sinusitis.

Normal for you may not really be normal at all. You may have learned to live with this condition, and consider it just a part of life that you will have repeated sinus infections. Sinus infections that require a trip to the doctor several times a year, a course of antibiotics several times a year, and then, the acceptance of a lower level of quality of life that leaves you fatigued and irritable, but still able to perform your functions in the work place and at home

Chronic Sinusitis

The usual symptoms of the common cold appear: the sore throat, headache, hoarseness, cough and the nasal congestion. This is followed by the postnasal drip of sinusitis but now there is more. Increased sensitivity to allergens with repeated allergic responses to either food or inhalants. There is a chronic low-grade infection and intermittent sinus infections, as well as a persistent loss of the sense of taste or smell, or both. The condition doesn't last for five to seven days, it doesn't last for a couple of weeks, it lasts for months.

If you have wondered how it can get worse than acute sinusitis—you have your answer. A chronic, persistent low-grade infection with periodic recurrences of acute sinusitis.

Perhaps you take a course of antibiotics and

then find that the infection returns in a couple of weeks after the completion of the regimen. Perhaps you never feel really well. Maybe you have had a sinus surgery and that still doesn't get rid of the postnasal drip. These are the symptoms of chronic sinusitis.

Have you become increasingly sensitive to inhalants, such as cigarette smoke, auto fumes, dry air, perfumes?

You may have chronic sinusitis.

Has it has been months, perhaps years, since you can really recall not having a headache, the loss of your sense of smell or taste, the constant postnasal drip down the back of the throat, the chronic fatigue, perhaps the continual ache-all-over feeling that accompanies a persistent low-grade infection?

You may have chronic sinusitis.

If there is any good news, it is that a person with chronic sinusitis is not usually as sick or as miserable as a person with acute sinusitis.

The Number One Health Problem in the U.S.

No one should be surprised to hear sinusitis is number one chronic health complaint in the U.S.

The National Center for Health Statistics, in *National Health Interview Survey of 1994,* lists *four* respiratory conditions among the ten most common chronic diseases afflicting Americans today:

1. Sinusitis
2. Arthritis
3. Hypertension
4. Allergic rhinitis (hay fever)
5. Orthopedic impairment
6. Heart disease
7. Hearing impairment
8. Chronic bronchitis
9. Asthma
10. Migraine headache

These four chronic respiratory conditions—sinusitis, allergic rhinitis, bronchitis and asthma all affect a part of the same tract: the respiratory tract.

It should not be forgotten that the nose is the body's first line of defense against infectious agents entering the respiratory tract and, as such, the nose and its mucous membrane need to be in good health to ward against disease.

Frequently, these common respiratory conditions occur either together, or one after the other.

Asthma

The word *asthma* comes from the Greek work for "panting," and this refers to the attacks of shortness of breath. The recurrent spasms of respiratory difficulty, characterized by a wheezing type of breathing, makes asthma the most frightening and life-threatening of common respiratory conditions. It affects the small airways, the bronchioles, and causes swelling of the respiratory mucosa lining the airway, increases and thickens the secretions into the airway and causes the smooth muscle lining the bronchiolar walls to contract. The three obstructive changes—swelling of mucosa, increase of secretions and muscle contraction—make it very difficult for air to pass through. This difficulty in breathing results in an audible wheeze, a cough, a constricted chest and congested lungs. The airway becomes hyper-responsive to airborne allergens, pollutants, and both cold and dry air.

Fifteen million Americans suffer from asthma, the chronic obstructive condition of the bronchial tubes. The incidence and severity of asthma seems to be growing worldwide. In the U.S., the number of asthma cases rose seventy percent from 1980 to 1989, and the death rate is rising eight percent a year. It is the most common chronic pediatric illness, afflicting more than three million children and resulting in approximately eight million missed school days each year. Allergist Allan Weinstein says that it is the most common reason for children being admitted to the hospital.

In parts of the South Bronx, asthma is so common that doctors in the area's main hospital,

Lincoln, say they have received thirteen thousand visits a year for asthma for the past several years. Researchers have identified a number of inner-city characteristics they believe contribute to the epidemic, the most important being indoor air pollution.

Persons whose asthma is precipitated only by allergenic exposure to airborne pollens and molds, house dust, animal danders—those with *extrinsic* asthma—account for about ten to twenty percent of the adult asthmatic population. By contrast, thirty to fifty percent of adult asthmatics are *intrinsic* asthmatics, meaning their symptomatic episodes appear to be triggered by non-allergenic factors (infection, irritants, emotions) interacting with a sensitive airway. For a great number of asthmatics, both allergic and non-allergic factors appear to play significant triggering roles.

Secondary factors can perpetuate asthmatic attacks and may profoundly influence the severity and frequency of these attacks. Such secondary factors can include endocrine changes (menopause, pregnancy, puberty, menstruation), environmental changes (humidity and temperature), as well as exposure to noxious fumes (paints, chemicals, smoke). These secondary factors precipitate symptoms by upsetting the delicate balance maintained between the individual and his environment.

A study of asthma by Dutch and American researchers dispels the myth that symptoms of this sometimes fatal lung disease abate in adulthood. Although many children with the mildest symptoms of asthma do outgrow the disease, it is clear that those with moderate or severe asthma usually do not.

However, it may not be inevitable that infants born to parents with a history of an allergic disorder such as asthma will develop symptoms. A study reported in the June 1992 *Lancet* confirms that avoiding exposure to allergens in the first year of life can help prevent or delay childhood allergies and asthma. According to Gary Rachelefsky, director of the Allergy Research Foundation, the development of asthma can be prevented through both food and environmental controls. He believes if such a regimen postpones asthmatic symptoms for the first year, the benefits would be enormous to the continued good health of any child.

The number of women suffering from asthma has risen sharply in the past decade. A number of theories have been put forward to explain the trend. Doctors are diagnosing asthma more than they did in the past, when it was classified with other lung-related problems. Women's increased participation in sports may also be a culprit because strenuous physical activity can trigger attacks.

Similarly, because more women are working outside the home, they may be increasingly exposed to the allergens that thrive in the air-conditioning and carpets of tightly sealed offices.

Worldwide, asthma appears to be on the increase, possibly as a result of air pollution or other environmental changes.

Throughout the 1980s, when death rates for nearly every childhood disease except AIDS were on the decline, deaths from childhood asthma were on the rise. The death rate in 1989 was nearly double what it was in 1979. Most of the 5000-plus people who die of asthma annually are elderly, but the death rate in the 5-14 age group has been increasing most rapidly, by about ten percent a year over the past decade. The black/white gap in deaths has also been widening: blacks were twice as likely as whites to die from asthma in 1979, and three times as likely in 1989. According to Robinson Fulwood of the National Health, Lung and Blood Institute's National Asthma Education Program, the rates are disproportionate because most minority children live in urbanized areas, are subjected to more environmental pollutants, and have limited access to health care.

A study by a team at the University of Washington in Seattle provided evidence that links wood stove smoke to respiratory illness. Jane Q. Koenig and coworkers studied the lung-function tests of 327 children. They found that in two Seattle-area elementary schools located in a valley which formed a bowl trapping the wood smoke, asthmatic children had a nine percent drop in their breathing ability during the cold winter months when wood stoves were used in this area.

Frank Speizer, at the Harvard School of Public Health in Boston, and a team of epidemiologists interviewed students from a Boston-area high school and compared their rates of illness to controls at a neighboring school. Significantly higher numbers of students at the Boston-area school reported experiencing such health problems as chronic coughing, wheezing, and chest illnesses. Speizer notes this school was well known for the so-called Sick Building Syndrome, and the types of illnesses reported were those typically associated with stagnant air containing high amounts of dust, carbon dioxide and chemicals.

Researchers who studied army trainees for four years, in four different training camps, found the incidence of respiratory disease was forty-five percent higher among those housed in modern barracks than in the living in barracks built in the 1940s and 1950s. The researchers believe that the difference is due to modern heating and cooling systems, which recirculate about ninety-five percent of the air in the buildings to save energy. The older buildings recycled only fifty percent to sixty percent of indoor air.

It appears that allergies play a dual role in causing asthma and in triggering individual episodes. When the lungs are overstimulated by viral infections, allergens, or pollutants, the body activates the immune system, causing airways to swell and muscles surrounding the airways to contract, cutting off air flow. Once asthma begins, it establishes a feedback loop that may require only general irritants to trigger an attack.

Researchers at the University of Wisconsin Medical School investigated the link between viruses and asthma. They found forty percent of children develop wheezing when they are afflicted by a respiratory infection, and many adults state their asthma emerged during a viral infection. The virus that causes croup is the most likely to induce wheezing in infants and young children, whereas a member of the rhinovirus family is linked to adult asthma. According to William Busse, the school's chief of allergy and clinical immunology, the allergic reactions a virus induces, coupled with the virus's effect on lung tissue, makes an asthmatic condition worse among those with colds.

There is hardly any doubt that sinusitis and asthma are interrelated. A 1989 study noted that more than two-thirds of patients with mild to severe asthma showed abnormalities in the sinuses when examined by X-ray. The same study reported that asthmatic children with moderate to severe sinus abnormalities were improved with treatment to alter their sinus condition, in addition to the treatment of the asthma.

The National Jewish Center for Immunology and Respiratory Medicine in Denver, which treats asthmatics whose asthma is poorly controlled or who depend on cortisone to control their condition, described many patients who improved greatly and were able to decrease their steroid requirements after treatment of their sinuses.

At one time, attention was focused on bronchospasm (due to smooth muscle contraction) as the major contributor to the airway obstruction. More recently, it is understood that asthma, particularly in its chronic form, is truly an inflammatory disease of the airways. Typically, asthmatics with an active condition have hyper-responsive or hypoactive airways, manifested as an exaggerated bronchoconstrictor response to many different stimuli. The degree of hyper-responsiveness is closely linked to the extent of the inflammation.

A bronchial asthma attack is characterized by: bronchi are plugged with thick, tenacious, slightly cloudy mucus; bronchial walls are constricted because of spasm or increased bronchial smooth muscle tone and thickening (as a result of acute inflammation and swelling); hyperactive mucous glands; and hyperinflation of the alveoli, alveolar ducts and respiratory bronchioles.

During an acute asthmatic attack, air movement is impaired during expiration because of the constriction of the swollen bronchial tubes filled with excess secretions. Characteristically a wheeze occurs and expiration is prolonged because air is being forced through these constricted bronchi. The lungs are hyper-extended and, as the attack worsens, a temporary emphysema-like situation occurs, with air trapped in and ballooning out the tiny alveoli. This air trapping occurs after air enters the alveoli because the bronchial tubes narrow during the effort to expel the air. The trapped air distends the tiny alveolar walls and weakens them.

In allergic forms of asthma the local bronchial reaction is caused by an antigen-antibody combination reaction. In addition to the tissue changes already mentioned, increased capillary permeability takes place and an increased number of a particular kind of blood cell, which is meant to combat invaders, appears on the scene, adding to the congestion.

Asthmatic attacks are sudden and vary in frequency, intensity and duration. Most commonly they are of short duration and between attacks you may be asymptomatic. A few symptoms may persist, especially upon exertion or during extremes of emotion.

Attacks frequently begin suddenly, without warning, when you are at rest. Typically, you might feel a sudden shortness of breath and the feeling of suffocating or drowning.

The typical response is to stand up and lean forward, devoting most energy to breathing. Each expiration will be prolonged; wheezing is most pronounced during the expiration and can often be heard at some distance. Respirations are difficult, but the rate of frequency is normal. Cough and sputum production commonly occur. Quite often termination of the attack is indicated by severe coughing and expectoration of thick, tenacious sputum followed by a feeling of relief and then a clearing of the airways.

During severe attacks the chest is markedly distended and the neck veins bulge, due to increased pressure caused by the air trapped in the lungs. Profuse perspiration often occurs as a result of increased nerve response, indicating the stress to which you are being subjected and the effort being expended. Rapid heart rate, audible wheezes are both often present. Because of sweating and increased insensible water loss from the lungs, variable degrees of dehydration may occur with prolonged episodes. You may feel more comfortable sitting upright or even leaning forward, using accessory muscles to breathe.

In more severe episodes, you may be unable to speak more than a few words without stopping for breath. Fatigue and severe distress are evident in rapid, shallow and ineffective respiratory movements. Cyanosis (blue-tinged skin) will become evident as the attack worsens. Confusion and lethargy may indicate the onset of progressive respiratory failure. After a severe attack your chest may be quite sore.

Symptoms may subside in less than hour or may persist for several hours.

Asthma worsens at night, tightening the airways as you sleep. In individuals without asthma, there is about a five percent change in lung function overnight, the asthmatic's change in lung function is twenty percent. In a survey conducted at Harvard Medical School of 8,000 people, it was found that three out of four with asthma had at least one nighttime attack each week. An even more alarming statistic is that most asthma deaths occur during the night, and approximately nine-tenths of them occur between 10 PM and 7 AM.

During the day, two naturally occurring asthma hormones keep you breathing freely: adrenaline, which dilates the airways, and corticosteroids, which act as anti-inflammatories. During sleep, however, the levels of these hormones decrease—your airways tighten—with an increased tendency to spasm at night.

If symptoms persist for several days, it is possible that *status asthmaticus* can develop. Status asthmaticus is a condition of acute bronchospasm and is not relieved by conventional bronchodilator therapy. It is a serious, exhausting condition which needs immediate medical intervention.

All asthma attacks, of whatever amount of severity, are serious, frightening and exhausting experiences.

Asthma is diagnosed from: (1) a history of recurrent paroxysmal attacks of difficult or labored breathing, cough, wheezing and the production of mucoid sputum; (2) a family or personal history of allergy; (3) prolonged exhalation with wheezing noises; and (4) eosinophils (a particular type of white blood cell) in the sputum or the blood.

The Merck Manual describes the staging of the severity of an acute asthma attack as follows:

I (mild)—mild dyspnea (labored breathing), diffuse wheezes, adequate air exchange.

II (moderate)—respiratory distress at rest, hyperpnea (abnormal increase in the depth and rate of breathing), use of accessory muscles to breathe, marked wheezing.

III (severe)—marked respiratory distress, cyanosis (blue-tinged skin), use of accessory muscles to breathe, marked wheezes or absent breath sounds, a variant pulse.

IV (respiratory failure)—severe respiratory distress, lethargy, confusion, se of accessory muscles to breathe, a variant pulse.

David Levin, professor of medicine at the University of Oklahoma Health Sciences Center, notes the public still believes several myths about asthma. Among these misconceptions are asthma is never fatal, only children have it, children with asthma should not be as active as their peers, people with asthma are emotionally unstable and asthma leads to emphysema, which appears to be an entirely separate disease.

Asthma can occur secondarily to a variety of stimuli, although the underlying mechanisms responsible for the attacks are unknown; inherited or acquired imbalances of those chemicals in the bloodstream responsible for airway diameter—which changes automatically when oxygen needs change—have been implicated. Some individuals who manifest such imbalances can have bronchoconstriction at subclinical levels but present no symptoms.

Changes in the pulmonary airways contribute

to a special kind of inflammation characteristic of asthma. These changes lead to airway obstruction in varying degrees and this obstruction provides ventilation that is not uniform. Continued blood flow to some areas of low ventilation then leads to an imbalance, resulting in a deficiency of arterial blood oxygen, which is almost always present in attacks severe enough to require medical attention. As an asthma attack progresses, the individual's capacity to compensate by increased ventilation of the unobstructed areas of the lungs is further impaired by more extensive airway narrowing and muscular fatigue, caused by the increasingly difficult work of breathing.

Stress can trigger the hyperreactive bronchial trees of asthmatics to begin responding. We ordinarily think of stress as emotional or work-related, but the stress placed on the bronchial system of the asthmatic can include a great variety of things: viral respiratory infections; exercise; emotional upsets; nonspecific factors (e.g., changes in barometric pressure or temperature); inhalation of cold air or such irritants as gasoline fumes, fresh paint and other noxious odors, or cigarette smoke; as well as exposure to allergens that are specific to that individual.

It is now recognized that asthma is a hereditary immune system disorder that is sometimes linked to allergies and stressors. The asthmatic needs to be aware of what stressors can precipitate the reaction of their hyperactive respiratory system in order to avoid upsetting the delicate balance between the individual and the asthma-causing environment.

Allergic Rhinitis

Swelling and inflammation of the mucous membrane is the most common symptom of allergic rhinitis. The other most common symptoms are sneezing and itching, with a clear, thin mucus drainage. Often the eyes are included, with itching, watering and constant tearing.

Pollen

Approximately 27 million Americans suffer from allergic rhinitis or hay fever, and the largest group of these sufferers are sensitive to pollen from trees, grass or ragweed. The symptoms can be seasonal. Pollen from trees is most abundant from March to May; pollen from grasses from May to July; ragweed from August to October. This may vary, of course, depending upon the location of the trees and grass, as well as the weather, which determines just when pollen occurs. While these three substances cause the most trouble for the most people, there are many other substances that can cause allergic rhinitis on a year-round basis.

Dust mites

Dust mites, microscopic insects that live wherever dust collects, are high on the list of offenders. They live on shed human skin cells and leave droppings that are similar in size to pollen and can be inhaled. Dust mites are the main reason many allergists recommend carpeting and drapes be removed from the homes of any one who suffers severely from allergic rhinitis or asthma.

Mold

Mold spores can grow on food, furniture, air conditioning units, crops, grass and dead leaves, and occur in sizes small enough to be inhaled.

Pets

Cats are frequent causes of allergic reactions in those sensitive to animal dander. Cats naturally and regularly shed tiny flakes of skin. These flakes mix with fur and the cat's saliva, which contains a protein called Fel d1. This mix of skin, fur and saliva becomes airborne when the animal scratches. It can rub off to your skin and clothing when you pet or hold a cat, or when you sit on furniture where a cat has been.

Washing a cat weekly with lukewarm distilled water may make it safe for the allergic person to live with a cat. After 3 to 8 months, the cat will stop producing Fel d1—in essence, creating a non-allergic cat. Washing with distilled water doesn't harm the pet or remove too much oil from its fur.

Bathing a cat can be less traumatic for both you and the cat with a little preparation. Place three or four warm towels (put them in the dryer, or the oven for a few minutes) by a comfortable place where you can dry the cat in your lap after the bath. Place a towel within easy reach of the bath area and one in the bottom of the sink so the cat can feel there is something to grip with his hind feet rather than sliding around on a slippery surface. Don't begin to wet the cat until you are sure the water temperature is comfortable.

If you are using a sink, place the hind paws in the sink and the front paws on the drainboard. Remember, the water is not going to hurt, the cat is just fearful of the unknown. Leave the head until last, it can always be wiped down with a damp washcloth later. Talk to the cat in a soothing voice, with your face close to his, letting him know you are doing something good for him. He can understand the tone in your voice, and be calmed by the sound. The first couple of baths, make it a quick process, until he begins to understand it won't hurt. After bathing, place the cat on your lap for drying. It isn't necessary to get him completely dry, as long as it is a warm day or the room is well-heated.

Other pets, including dogs and birds can cause allergic reactions. Cleaning the bedding and cages of these pets can go a long way to keeping the allergens they produce from becoming airborne.

Food

There are numerous foods that cause allergic reactions in sensitive individuals. Some of the most frequent allergens are: dairy products, wheat, rye, corn, citrus, eggs and artificial food colorings. Elimination diets are the method used to detect food sensitivities. In allergic individuals, it is often found that these items can be slowly added back into the diet, up to a point of tolerance.

Some physicians believe that almost anyone can become sensitive to a food—particularly a favorite one—just by overload: eating the same thing day after day, as many people do. If food sensitivity creates a problem, it is best to eat a variety of foods, rather than a limited menu.

Allergic rhinitis with its continual nasal congestion can be a contributory cause of sinus infections.

Bronchitis

Acute bronchitis (infectious) or chronic bronchitis (inflammation) is often the result of a common cold or other viral infection of the nasopharynx, throat, or tracheobronchial tree, often with a secondary bacterial infection. Exposure to air pollutants, and possibly chilling, fatigue and malnutrition, are predisposing or contributory factors. Recurrent attacks often complicate chronic bronchopulmonary diseases; they suggest a focus of infection such as chronic sinusitis, allergy or, in children, hypertrophied tonsils and adenoids.

Acute irritative bronchitis may be caused by occupational exposure to dust or toxic fumes, tobacco smoke, mineral or vegetable dusts of various kinds, fumes from certain volatile chemicals or other noxious inhalants.

Sinobronchitis is an infection of both the sinuses and the lungs caused by the postnasal drainage of infected mucus into the lungs. In addition to the usual symptoms of a sinus infection, there is a persistent productive cough, accompanied by yellow mucus, which is frequently more pronounced in the morning hours.

Asthmatic bronchitis is bronchitis with asthma. Breathing is extremely difficult, and the wheezing, coughing and laborious breathing is complicated by an infection of the bronchi, the two large tubes that branch off into the lungs from the windpipe.

In chronic bronchitis, excessive mucus is secreted by the inflamed respiratory mucosa lining the bronchi. According to the American Lung Association, to be diagnosed with chronic bronchitis you must have a productive cough, in which thick white mucus is produced, for at least three months, recurring for at least two consecutive years. Chronic bronchitis is often accompanied by wheezing, shortness of breath, weakness and weight loss.

Major Contributory Factors

While viruses and bacteria are major causes of sinusitis and bronchitis, there are contributory factors that can increase the likelihood of your having a respiratory ailment or developing a chronic condition. Thirty-five percent of the American population—approximately 100 million individuals—suffers from some type of chronic respiratory ailment: sinusitis, asthma, allergy or bronchitis.

Tobacco and secondhand smoke

In 1990 the Centers for Disease Control counted more than 400,000 deaths, including of course, lung cancer, directly attributable to tobacco products. 1996 has brought about the most notorious exposure of the tobacco industry to date, with company insiders acknowledging the part that their industry has played in downplaying the role of their products in these deaths.

Industrial exhaust and automobile exhausts

The Clean Air Act, passed in 1970, was intended to provide air-pollution control by the Environmental Protection Agency. Although this agency has identified hundreds of hazards in the air and has passed countless laws in an effort to reduce them, deaths from chronic lung diseases such as asthma, bronchitis, lung cancer, emphysema and tuberculosis are on the rise.

Some of this legislation includes "employee trip reduction" laws (an attempt to force twelve million solo commuters out of their cars in the smoggiest cities); mandating the sale of cleaner-burning cars and selling reformulated gasoline to meet higher emission standards; reaching accords with motorboat-engine manufacturers to voluntarily reduce smog-producing hydrocarbon and nitrogen oxide emissions.

Chemical pesticides

While most of us do not work regularly with pesticides, they are difficult to avoid. Their use on food products and in the environment (routine spraying of lawns and trees in urban areas and on farm crops in rural areas) makes them a part of everyday life whether we want them or not.

Many of the thirty-six chemical pesticides most commonly used in backyards have been connected to serious health problems. Results of a recent study at the University of North Carolina in Chapel Hill, for example, indicated that children whose yards were treated with pesticides were four times more to develop certain soft-tissue cancers.

A study by the International Rice Research Institute cast doubts on the value of pesticides. The report of this institute shows that both farmers and the community exaggerate the threat posed by pests to crops, while ignoring the health and economic costs of their application. They suggest that conserving the natural predators of crop pests consistently has the highest net benefits.

The *New York Times* recently reported that after decades of battling locusts and grasshoppers with toxic chemicals, scientists are developing a new generation of natural pesticides such as fungi and other natural enemies. They are being introduced into crops nationwide and are expected to be not only less hazardous to the environment but more selective in reaching their targets.

According to Jerry McLaughlin, professor of pharmacognosy at Purdue University, a biodegradable pesticide made from the bark of the paw paw tree has been shown to be effective against a wide variety of insect pests.

Government scientists have been releasing promising new research of agricultural chemicals that break down into harmless substances within a few days of application. Richard Dybus, the executive director of research at Merck, believes that biodegradable agricultural chemicals and microbial control of pests will take on a greater role in pest control in the future.

The Environmental Protection Agency has issued Working Protection Standards, and farmers will be held accountable for implementing these standards. The EPA has a voluntary program with the states to issue verification cards to individuals who receive appropriate training for working with pesticides. It gives states flexibility in administering the program but violation of the WPS regulations carries both criminal and civil penalties.

While none of us care to have bugs in our food or our homes, we should encourage legislation that reduces the use of toxic chemicals in our environment, supplanting these chemicals with less harsh and hazardous means.

For individual gardens, there are numerous books available which describe common plants that can be used as organic pesticides for fighting insects and diseases in the home garden. Citrus oil, garlic, marigolds, hot peppers, petunias, quackgrass, and tomatoes all can be used as both compost and insect deterrents.

Radon

Radon, a radioactive gas, is the product of the natural decay of uranium found in rocks and in the earth's crust. It is found in all buildings and it seeps into them through holes and cracks. Radon is an odorless and colorless gas, and most air cleaners do not remove it from the air.

The U.S. Environmental Protection Agency estimates that of the 140,000 lung cancer deaths in the U.S. each year, about 20,000 are radon-related. The EPA contends that many of those deaths could be avoided by reducing radon levels and cessation of smoking.

The Centers for Disease Control and Prevention, and the American Lung Association, contend that radon causes thousands of preventable lung cancer deaths annually, and when combined with smoking, can be an especially serious health risk.

Salt Lake City-based engineering consultant Vern Rogers and his colleagues analyzed radon's diffusion through samples of residential concrete. They found that molecules of radon gas passed through two- to four-inch thick samples of concrete. Although no studies looked at the effects of this gas on the sinuses, something this hazardous to the lungs cannot be beneficial to any other body structures.

Sulfur dioxide emissions

Produced by coal-burning power plants and smelters, the Clean Air Act has brought tougher legislation to bear on those industries producing these noxious emissions.

Epidemiologist Bart Ostro, of the California Department of Health Services in Berkeley, and colleagues analyzed data collected in the north-central Los Angeles area. Their study, which focused on 320 generally healthy, nonsmoking men and women, indicated that upper respiratory problems arose more often on the haziest days or days with the highest peaks in smog ozone. Severe smog also coincided with more lower respiratory problems among participants whose homes lacked air conditioners. Russell Sherwin and colleagues at the University of Southern California in Los Angeles detected signs of subtle, yet fairly extensive damage, in the lungs of eighty-five Los Angeles residents (ages 14 to 25) who had died in homicides or traffic accidents, indicating that severe smog affects everyone.

Another study, conducted by George Thurston of the New York University Medical Center's Department of Environmental Medicine in New York, supports the idea that acute respiratory ailments are more prevalent when air pollution levels are high. These researchers tracked daily concentrations of acid aerosols and ground-level ozone in New York City, Albany, and the Buffalo/Rochester area during the summer months of two years in the late 1980s. Their finds suggest that acid aerosols exacerbate the effects of ozone on the lung lining and that residents of urban centers suffer more from air pollution effects than suburban residents, despite similar exposures.

Carbon monoxide

Carbon monoxide cannot be seen, smelt or tasted, but it kills approximately 250 Americans a year and sends another 5,000 to the hospital by reducing the blood's ability to carry oxygen. It is a poisonous gas produced by the incomplete combustion of fuel, and any fuel-burning appliance can be a source.

The death of tennis player Vitas Gerulaitis in 1994 drew attention to this deadly gas. His death was attributed to a malfunctioning pool heater that vented into a pool-side bungalow where Gerulaitis was staying.

Automobile inspections by many states have been effective in reducing this airborne source of pollution by discovering leaks in exhaust systems or incomplete burning of automobile fuels; an annual inspection of any fuel burning appliance by a qualified service technician, plus the installation of a carbon monoxide detector can assist in the reduction of this hazard.

While the EPA is working to reduce these hazards and monitor them more carefully, there is a burgeoning black market in chlorofluorocarbons (CFCs), in which importers bring tons of the chemicals from Europe into ports in the U.S. That black market topped 22,000 tons of CFCs in 1994, according to export/import documents analyzed by Ozone Action, an environmental group.

In 1995, Republican Representative John T. Doolittle of California introduced a bill to postpone a ban on the production of CFCs despite the EPA's commitment to an estimated $53 billion phaseout of CFCs and all of the other chemicals implicated in ozone depletion.

The EPA estimates that the cost of complying with environmental mandates will exceed $32 billion by the year 2000. While many critics—primarily economists—share with most Americans the goal of a cleaner environment, they contend that environmental mandates often impose enormous costs on society, and they are fearful that the efforts by local governments to obtain revenues

Section III

Treating Sinusitis

Sinusitis is an inflammatory process in the paranasal sinuses due to viral, bacterial, and fungal infections or allergic reactions.

Acute sinusitis is generally caused by streptococci, pneumococci or staphylococci bacteria which are everywhere, and are readily transmittable from one individual to another. A sinus infection is usually the result of an acute viral respiratory tract infection. In approximately twenty-five percent of cases of chronic maxillary sinusitis, it is secondary to a dental infection.

With any upper respiratory tract infection, the swollen nasal mucous membrane obstructs the draining of the paranasal sinus, and the oxygen in the sinus is absorbed into the blood vessels in the mucous membrane. This results in a relative negative pressure in the sinus which is painful. If this vacuum is maintained, the resulting fluid from the mucous membrane fills the sinus, where it serves as a medium for bacterial growth. The immune system goes to work to combat this condition with an outpouring of serum and blood cells known as leukocytes, whose job it is to combat such infectious gatherings. The result is a very painful positive pressure within the obstructed sinus.

Upon examination, the area over the involved sinus may be tender and swollen. Pain may occur in the cheeks or in the teeth. There may be a frontal headache. A pain behind and between the eyes is often described as a "splitting headache." There usually is fatigue. Fever and/or chills suggest the infection has spread beyond the sinuses.

The mucosa of the nose is red and swollen; there may be yellow or green pus. When examined with an illuminating scope, the frontal and maxillary sinuses may be opaque. Nasal endoscopy is a procedure performed by both allergists and ear, nose and throat specialists, using a rod lens telescope that is inserted into the nasal cavity. This permits visualization of the interior of the nose, including the opening of the ostia. It is performed in the office using topical anesthesia. This procedure can pinpoint pathological changes in the tissue, assist in making a correct diagnosis, and can be used to obtain samples of pus for culture. This is the most accurate method of pinpointing the actual bacteria causing the infection—far more accurate than a nasal swab—and will make it possible to identify the proper antibiotic for the infection, rather than using a broad spectrum antibiotic. However, most individuals with sinusitis are seen by their primary care physicians (in the case of HMOs), and by internists and pediatricians, and are usually not referred on to a specialist until the condition is so continuous and repetitive that specialized examination is deemed necessary.

X-rays are usually taken by these specialists to reliably define the sites and the degree of involvement. X-rays are often required to exclude abscesses of the teeth.

Antibiotics

The aim of conventional therapy is to improve drainage and to control any infection. However, sinusitis is not a simple infection to treat. Seldom is the bacteria that caused the infection identified. Physicians usually select a broad-spectrum antibiotic in an effort to cover a wide range of possible pathogens. Because antibiotics are taken orally and then absorbed into the blood stream, it usually takes several days for the effects to be felt.

Drainage improvement is tried with a combination of steam inhalation (which dilutes the thickened mucus) and decongestants, antihistamines and vasoconstrictors. Unfortunately, one of the side effects of prolonged use of decongestants is a "rebound" effect. That is, the decongestant attempts to dry up the mucus by thickening it and, as a result, the membrane produces more mucus in an effort to keep itself at the proper moisture balance. The same is true of antihistamines, which shrink the membrane and thicken the mucus, preventing it from draining.

Amoxicillin is presently the drug of choice of most physicians, unless there is an allergy to penicillin. Adults should expect a definite improvement in approximately four to five days. Children usually respond more rapidly than adults, within approximately forty-eight hours. The standard instructions are to take the antibiotic for ten days. If individuals do not comply with the regimen, the infection often remains, to reoccur shortly.

Despite compliance, approximately ten percent of individuals with a sinus infection will not be cured by antibiotics. When this happens, the next step the physician takes is to prescribe a different antibiotic. The second-choice antibiotics have a broader spectrum of efficacy. Even then, a number of these patients are still not cured, or the infection recurs shortly thereafter.

Often, it is only after repeated infections or reoccurrences—with the fatigue, illness and constant drainage—that the family practitioner will refer someone out to the specialist for a further diagnostic evaluation with the X-ray, CT scan or nasal endoscopy. Unfortunately, this process of recurrences and return visits to the physician can drag on for months or sometimes even longer without any real relief from the condition.

In recent years, there has been a great deal of publicity given to the over-prescription of antibiotics as a cure-all, as a result of which we have produced new strains of antibiotic-resistant bacteria, called super germs.

According to the Centers for Disease Control and Prevention, 19,000 hospital patients die annually from antibiotic-resistant infections, and another 58,000 people die because of complications attributable to bacterial infections. Many individuals who suffer from chronic sinusitis are still sick because their sinuses are now infected with antibiotic-resistant bacteria. For these people, repeated treatment with antibiotics is useless.

Stuart B. Levy, MD, professor of medicine, molecular biology and microbiology, and Director of the Center for Adaptation Genetics and Drug Resistance at Tufts University School of Medicine, believes that up to fifty percent of all antibiotic use in the U.S. today is actually misuse; and some experts estimate that half of all prescriptions written are unnecessary. Why do doctors write them? Because the public wants to believe that antibiotics are a cure-all; they don't want to be sick, and think that the answer to every illness is an antibiotic. Some physicians feel that to write a prescription for an unnecessary antibiotic is necessary to retain the patient, or to just "do something" to make the individuals feel that they are being given some kind of help.

Dr. Levy, in his book *The Antibiotic Paradox,* states that the same antibiotics that prevent bacteria from killing people also breed antibiotic-resistant super germs. Bacteria continue to evolve, changing their form in an effort to survive. Livestock are routinely given antibiotics in their feed to prevent infections. Today's milk may contain as many as eighty different antibiotics. The human habit of stopping a course of antibiotics as soon as the person is feeling better also contributes to this undesirable growth. It is necessary to take the entire course of the medicine (that is the ten or fourteen days, or whatever length of time for which it is prescribed) because the bacteria are in differing stages of their own growth cycle, and unless every single germ is killed, reinfection can occur as soon as the medication is stopped. Bacteria have an outer shell, and the antibiotic must enter this shell at a particular time in the youth of the bacteria. If the bacteria live beyond a certain point, the shell becomes impenetrable, thus allowing the bacteria to live and reproduce, living to re-infect the body.

There is growing evidence that antibiotics interfere with the body's immune system, weakening the ability to fight off other invading bacteria. Over 1,000 antibiotics have been invented since penicillin was discovered in 1942. Scientists now believe more care should be taken in using existing antibiotics, rather than developing new ones. They suggest careful use may mean doctors should write fewer prescriptions, there should be less overuse and misuse of antibiotics in animal agriculture, and veterinarians should prescribe fewer antibiotics for pets. Thirty million pounds of antibiotics are used every year in the U.S. Bacteria have evolved by producing packages of genes that counteract each of the five main classes of antibiotics, and these packages are passed around, even between unrelated strains of bacteria.

Just fifty years after antibiotics revolutionized the practice of medicine, these "wonder drugs" are losing their edge. Some experts fear a return to the days when drugs were powerless against major killers, such as tuberculosis and pneumonia. Pharmaceutical companies have revived their antibiotic research and development programs in response to the emergence of antibiotic-resistant strains of pathogenic bacteria. Preliminary reports on several new antibiotics were presented at the 35th Interscience Conference on Anti-Microbial Agents and Chemotherapy held in September 1995. However, most of these new antibiotics will not be available for clinical use for at five to fifteen years.

Everyone who takes medications of any sort should be aware of the possible side effects or adverse effects of those medications. The PDR, or *Physicians' Desk Reference* is available in every pharmacy and every library, and a review of its pages ought to be a regular part of the homework of anyone taking any medication.

Some researchers believe that constant antibiotic treatments also destroy the friendly bacteria in our digestive tract, which allows for the overgrowth of Candida albicans, a single-celled fungi of the genus Candida—an organism which is normally present in the vagina and gastrointestinal tract. Most people harbor some of these microorganisms in their bodies at various times; problems arise when the fungi multiply out of control, usually in connection with some types of immune suppression. Stress, poor nutrition, HIV infection, diabetes, pregnancy, and the use of any medication, including birth control pills, can encourage yeast to thrive.

Dr. Stuart Berger, in his *Immune Power Diet,* states that one out of three people is allergic to common foods, and that these allergies disrupt the immune system, causing such maladies as infection, obesity, and aches and pains. Most allergists, however, believe that only one to two percent of the adult population has food allergies.

Dr. William Crook's *The Yeast Connection,* another book that claims a connection between diet and the immune system, asserts that people who have a high level of certain toxin-producing yeasts (i.e., Candida albicans) are likely to experience fatigue and depression, among other ailments. Crook recommends eliminating the foods yeast thrive on: sugar, honey, molasses, and other sugary items.

However, many in the mainstream nutrition community are skeptical of the claims of both of these authors.

Anyone taking a course of antibiotics should commit to taking the treatment for the entire duration prescribed in order to eradicate all the pathogens. In addition, it is necessary to take acidophilus powder or live culture yogurt in order to replenish the good bacteria which are in the intestines and are necessary for good health. Acidophilus powder or capsules can be purchased at the health food store, and live culture yogurt will state that is live on the outside of the container. Many yogurts found today in the grocery store are not live culture and have been flavored and sugared for taste, having very little dietary benefit other than perhaps a few grams of calcium.

Individuals who do not respond to antibiotics should be seen by a specialist for a diagnostic evaluation wit X-ray, CT scan or nasal endoscopy to see if there is the possibility of a physical obstruction of the sinuses.

Further, anyone with repeated sinus infections which no longer respond to antibiotic treatment might want to consider looking at fungi as being the culprit rather than a repeated viral infection.

Decongestants

Decongestants are readily available in familiar over-the-counter products. Most of these contain an antihistamine in combination with the decongestant. Decongestants are used to open the ostia and ducts of the sinus, in conjunction with an analgesic, to relieve the symptoms of head and nasal congestion: headache and facial pain. Some over-the-counter medications are aimed specifically at sinus conditions and have a name which designates them as such, such as Sinutab.

The most common ingredients in both prescription and over-the-counter decongestants are pseudoephedrine, phenylpropanolamine, and phenylephrine. They all work to shrink swollen mucous membranes and reduce nasal and sinus congestion. Many products contain these decongestants in various combinations. Others contain a pain reliever or analgesic, or an expectorant or cough suppressant as well. Most of the by-prescription decongestants or expectorants contain higher doses of the named three medications, or are long-acting. Other than that, they are very similar to the over-the-counter products.

Decongestant Nasal Sprays

These medications are recommended for those with severe sinus headache and nasal congestion. A word of caution—they can be addictive.

Using a nasal spray decongestant for more than three or four consecutive days can lead to a type of dependence. According to David Fairbanks of the Ear, Nose & Throat Medical Group of Washington, D.C., overuse can cause the body's natural mechanism for controlling nasal congestion to stop working properly, and then there is a rebound effect: as the decongestant effect wears off, the head and nasal congestion returns and you may feel worse than you did before. The usual response is to increase the usage, resulting in further rebound effect. These sprays contain chemicals that constrict the nasal blood vessels: as their effects wear off, the expansion of these vessels is often responsible for difficulty in breathing. After the vessels have expanded and contracted for several days, however, they become fatigued and swell to an even greater extent, prompting affected people to spray with increasing frequency. People who have used nasal sprays for prolonged periods may require medical intervention, such as an injection of cortisone or even surgery, to reduce the swelling of the nasal tissues.

If you find you are unable to discontinue the use of a decongestant nasal spray, you may have become dependent. Advise the physician treating you, so you may get some assistance.

Fairbanks recommends stopping the use of such nasal sprays, even though you may feel congested without them, sleeping with the head propped up, and exercising regularly to counteract the stuffiness that will follow for a few days. The use of an oral decongestant during the transition to nonuse of sprays may make the change more tolerable.

Use moisture, including a saline nasal spray, a humidifier, and inhale steam in a closed bathroom or by a vaporizer.

Antihistamines

These medications work by temporarily blocking

the action of histamine, the substance produced by the body in response to allergens or other irritants that can cause itching, sneezing, runny nose and eyes, and other symptoms.

Antihistamines are available both by prescription and over the counter. They are generally taken for hay fever and other allergies. They may also be used to treat coughs, motion sickness, sleeplessness, hives and the symptoms of Parkinson's disease. A common side effect is drowsiness, which presents little danger. Doctors should be notified at once if blurred vision, painful urination, severe tiredness, unsteadiness, hallucinations, shortness of breath, loss of consciousness or dryness of the mouth, nose or throat occurs. Children under six should not be given antihistamines without consulting a doctor, and the drug should not be taken by anyone taking antidepressants.

Men with enlarged prostates may find antihistamines, particularly the non-sedating types, cause urinary problems. They relax the bladder and constrict the sphincter muscle at the exit of the bladder, causing more difficulties in urinating.

In many states, driving under the influence of antihistamines carries the same penalties as first offense drunk driving. Skills most affected by antihistamines include motor coordination, speed of reaction, visual search, and critical tracking.

There are now some antihistamines available which do not cause drowsiness, but these are generally less effective than others.

Antitussives (cough suppressants)

Sometimes the sinus condition is accompanied by a cough (the body's natural reaction to congestion). If the cough interrupts sleep or is so persistent it is exhausting you, the doctor may recommend you not take the bedtime dose of decongestant, but instead, take a prescription cough suppressant in combination with a decongestant, an expectorant, or both. Many antitussives cause drowsiness and should not be used during waking hours.

If a cough suppressant is necessary for daytime, an over-the-counter one should be sufficient to suppress the cough and not cause drowsiness.

Analgesics (pain relievers)

Headache, facial pain or sore throat which often accompany sinusitis can usually be relieved with an over-the-counter pain medication. Aspirin relieves pain and reduces inflammation but can cause some stomach upset or be harmful to those with ulcers or bleeding difficulties. Ibuprofen relieves pain and reduces inflammation. Acetaminophen relieves pain but does not reduce inflammation.

Children should be given either baby aspirin or an acetaminophen product. However, if the child has a fever, a doctor should be consulted before any medicine is administered because there is always the possibility of Reye's syndrome, caused by salicate medications—a sometimes fatal condition.

Hydration

Moisture will relieve nasal and head congestion, headache, sinus pain and sore throat. It is effective in assisting thinning the thick, infected mucus in the sinuses, which restores the cilia to normal functioning.

Moist, warm air can be created in a closed bathroom by turning on the shower, or by using a vaporizer. Vaporizers are readily available in most drug stores or pharmacies, particularly those which sell baby products. Hot moist towels placed over the face can also be effective in producing moist warm air.

Most humidifiers are effective in producing moisture in an enclosed space.

Humidifiers should be cleaned thoroughly after each use by washing with white vinegar to prevent the formation of molds, which could create another problem if inhaled.

During an infection it is best to use the humidifier or the steam from the shower daily. There are preparations, such as eucalyptus oil or other aromatic oils which can be purchased at the health food store, which can be added to the unit to enhance the beneficial effects and will assist in relieving the sinus headache.

In the winter, many homes are relatively dry, particularly if the furnace is operating for a number of hours. It is recommended that you add a humidifier to the furnace if possible. If not, a pan of hot water set on top of a radiator will add moisture to the air. This is most important in the bedroom to keep the sinuses moist during the night while you are sleeping.

Medical supply stores may also have a ultra-sonic vaporizer. This delivers 100 percent water-saturated pressurized air at a temperature of 110°F directly into the nasal passages. An ultrasonic tranducer vibrates water into very tiny droplets, approximately 4 to 8 microns in size. These units are more expensive than ordinary vaporizers or steam inhalers but are more effective as a nasal decongestant, thus allowing the sinuses to drain better. For individuals with frequent sinus infections, it may be well worth the additional cost.

Saline Spray and Irrigation

Saline sprays wash out some of the mucus, bacteria and dust particles. They can reduce the pressure on sinuses as well by increasing drainage, and will aid in reducing the swelling in the nasal passages. Sprays and irrigations aid in relieving the discomfort of dry, encrusted nasal membranes, and will aid in decreasing the possibility of nose-bleeds, which are common for individuals with sinusitis.

Dr. David Fairbanks, MD, spokesperson for the American Academy of Otolaryngology told *Prevention Magazine* that it is best to use distilled or sterile water in these irrigations, so you don't inadvertently cause an infection if there is an open sore in your nose. The water should be at about body temperature, that is 98.6°F.

Commercial varieties of saline sprays are available in pharmacies. This is nothing more than salt water in a handy squeeze bottle.

You can make your own saline spray by mixing 1/3 teaspoon of non-iodized table salt and a pinch of baking soda in an 8-ounce glass of luke-warm bottled non-chlorinated distilled or sterile water. This solution is close to the pH and normal body salinity of the human. Plain tap water is not as comfortable for the inside of the nose and leaves the lining of the nose dryer than it was before, rather than increasing the comfort level of this tissue. This homemade product can be used in the nose with any kind of a spray bottle.

To use saline spray, close off one nostril, spray into the other while inhaling. Saline spray is non-addictive and can be used as frequently as needed.

Saline irrigation can decrease pain and is more effective than simple sprays because it takes the saline deeper into the nasal cavity.

Prepare your saline solution as described.

Fill a large ear syringe (available at pharmacies or medical supply houses, the kind that comes in earwax-removal kits) with the solution. Lean over the sink or the tub. Insert the syringe tip just inside the nostril and pinch the other nostril closed. Gently squeeze the bulb several times to instill the solution into the nose. Do not do this forcefully, as it is possible to force mucus and bacteria up into the sinuses. All you want to do is to create an environment wherein the mucus and bacteria are diluted in order to make it possible for the sinuses to be able to drain.

Allow the solution to run out of your nose. Do not be alarmed if some runs out of your mouth. Repeat this procedure in each nostril until the solution runs clear.

You can pour the water into your nostril with a nasal cup, sometimes called a netti pot, which looks like a tiny teapot. One source for nasal cups is the *Self-Care Catalog.* You can order by calling 1-800-345-3371.

There are also nasal irrigation attachments for Water Pic appliances available for purchase. These operate on the same principle as the ear syringe, but send the stream of saline solution into the nostril. Many people find this easier to use and more accurate in controlling the pressure of the solution entering the nose.

For irrigating the nostrils of very small children, insert ten to twenty drops of saline per nostril with an eye dropper. This should be done very gently and with a full explanation beforehand, as many children find this frightening and fear they will be unable to breathe. However, many children find the relief worth the momentary discomfort and soon cooperate with the procedure.

Dr. Fairbanks warns against forcing water through your nose. You could end up trading a stuffy nose for an ear infection. If your congestion is thick or is a different color than usual, you should go to your doctor instead of trying to treat yourself.

After the nostrils seem to be clear for the moment, you may use a decongestant nasal spray if that has been recommended by a physician, as the irrigation will make the spray more effective.

After irrigation and spraying, apply an antibiotic ointment or a nasal emollient to the inside of the nose.

It is important to hydrate the body from the inside also, in order to keep the mucus thinned and draining. Drink at least eight glasses of water daily. Avoid ice-cold drinks as well as caffeine, sugar and alcohol.

As with any other infection, rest. If possible, do not over-tax yourself until the infection is under control and you begin to feel better.

Otolaryngology Evaluation

If, after a number of courses of antibiotics, you have done all the other things recommended (including possibly some alternative medicine treatments) but you are still suffering, then it is probably time to be seen by an expert, an otolaryngologist. Most patients seen by these specialists in the ear, nose and throat have been suffering with their condition at least a year: some even longer.

An initial evaluation by an ear, nose and throat specialist will include a physical examination of the structure of the nose, throat and sinuses. After applying a topical decongestant to the inside of the nose, a bacterial culture will be taken using nasal endoscopy. This culture will be taken from the opening of the sinus ducts (the ostia) in order to identify the specific bacterium that is causing the repeated infection. Unfortunately, the bacteria that reside just inside the nose are not usually the same as those causing the infection in the sinuses.

After the culture growth is identified in the laboratory, the specialist will usually prescribe a specific antibiotic—one that is specific to that particular germ—rather than a broad spectrum antibiotic, which is what a general practitioner will ordinarily do (a scatter-gun approach to attacking the offending organism).

Additional diagnostic procedures might include a CT scan of the sinuses. This is to ensure that, after the course of the specific antibiotic, all lingering pockets of infection have been removed and are not lurking in some small space, waiting to re-infect once again. Additionally, nasal endoscopy will determine if there is any obstruction around the ostia. A nasal cystogram will be performed: a microscopic inspection of cells from the nasal mucous membrane. This will possibly be followed by a complete battery of skin and blood tests to identify possible allergies.

During this time, which usually includes a ten-day to two-week course of one of the specific antibiotics identified, you will be required to perform nasal irrigation as well as other treatments, such as decongestants, as deemed appropriate.

If this does not result in an improvement in the condition—meaning that there is infection still visible on CT scan or the infection reoccurs shortly after the completion of the course of this new antibiotic—further evaluation will become necessary. After that evaluation, you might be given an alternative antibiotic and then, possibly, surgery will be suggested as the next step toward a cure of the condition.

Surgery

The most common surgery is a bilateral middle antrostomy. This surgery, performed through an endoscope, widens the maxillary sinus ostia from two millimeters to about ten or twelve millimeters, greatly improving the draining from these structures.

If there is any obstruction of the opening of the sinus duct into the nasal passage, such as polyps, cysts, an enlarged or distorted nasal turbinate or a deviated septum, this will be corrected. However, cysts and polyps have been known to recur, and this possibility should be considered before opting for surgery.

Once popular procedures such as the naso-antral window, the Caldwell-Luc operation or ethmoidectomy are seldom performed any longer as they are simply not as effective, and many patients who have had these surgeries have found they might need additional surgery.

Endoscopic surgery is now widely available, and is a marked improvement over the previous procedures. It is performed on an outpatient basis with local anesthesia. Patients can expect to be out of work for about one week.

Treating Asthma

Asthma is a lung disease which is characterized by (1) airways obstruction that is usually reversible, either spontaneously or with treatment, (2) airways inflammation, and (3) increased airways responsiveness to a variety of stimuli.

Asthma attacks are characterized by edema and inflammation of the bronchial mucosal wall, narrowing of the large and small airways due to bronchial smooth muscle spasm, and tenacious mucus production which results in decreased ventilation of the tiny air sacs known as alveoli. Continued failure of ventilation leads to an imbalance in oxygen levels in the blood stream, causing the sufferer to strive to increase oxygen intake, worsening the condition.

The clinical care of the asthmatic is directed toward providing immediate relief from acute attacks, reducing chronic symptoms (wheezing, coughing, shortness of breath), and minimizing the frequency of attacks.

Long term care is directed at controlling the causes of the attacks, and may include treatment of infection, emotional disorders and allergies.

When specific allergens are identified as precipitating asthmatic attacks, possible ways should be found to avoid these allergens. For example, someone found to be allergic to eggs, chocolate or wheat must take steps to eliminate these foods from the diet, and that may include reading labels of everything purchased and asking specific questions when dining out at restaurants.

Foods asthmatics are often allergic to include milk, eggs, chocolate, wheat and shellfish.

Medicines asthmatics are often allergic to include aspirin, antibiotics and iodine preparations.

When disorders such as chronic sinusitis, nasal polyps, and tonsillitis are present and are believed to contribute to the attacks, these conditions should be treated appropriately. Currently tonsils and adenoids are less often removed than formerly because of their recognized importance in the functioning of the immune response.

If infection is believed to contribute to asthma attacks, care should be directed to preventing recurrent respiratory infections.

Vaccines against pneumonia and influenza should be given to most asthmatics to aid in the avoidance of these seasonal illnesses.

You must learn to avoid or minimize secondary factors that precipitate attacks, e.g., fatigue, emotional stress. For some, psychotherapy may be useful in helping to maintain an optimal state of mental well-being. Sometimes small amounts of tranquilizers or sedatives will help with relaxation and the feeling of calmness.

Observations of your activities immediately prior to an attack may be helpful in identifying factors that precipitate one. Such observations should be charted; this may be very helpful in preventing future attacks.

Adequate hydration is very important. Some attacks are precipitated by dehydration of the mucous membranes. The asthmatic should drink 8 to 10 glasses of water daily in order to ensure the proper moisture balance of all bodily tissues.

Changes in climate are sometimes recommended for the person with severe asthma who does not respond to usual medical treatment. However, permanent moves should not be made until a trial residence period proves beneficial. For some, it may be desirable to avoid fog, smog, and extremely cold weather. However, for many, the climate change might be offset by exposure to a new set of allergens which may be just as undesirable as the ones just left behind.

The goals in treating the asthmatic include:
During an acute attack:
> maintaining efficient respiratory function while relieving bronchial spasm and promoting expulsion of secretions.

Thereafter:
> maintaining pulmonary function as close to normal as possible;

> maintaining activity levels as close to normal as possible;

> preventing chronic symptoms (coughing or breathlessness);

> preventing recurrent flare-ups;

> avoiding adverse effects of medications.

The National Institutes of Health state that the objective in treating chronic asthma is management of the disease. As of the present, there is nothing that is considered a cure.

The general principles involved in managing chronic asthma include:
> preventing or reversing the airway inflammation

> tailoring the treatment regime to the individual. Specific therapy is governed by the severity of the disease, tolerance to medication and sensitivity to aller-

gens, both food and environmental.

recognizing specific triggers, associated conditions and any special problems.

known allergens and/or irritants must be reduced or eliminated. Colds, sinus infections, middle ear infections and allergic rhinitis can trigger an asthma attack or aggravate an existing one.

Anyone who has asthma should consider both influenza and pneumonococcal vaccination.

Pulmonary function studies should be done regularly, to evaluate the baseline condition, as well as to keep updated on the continued lung functioning abilities.

Medications should be evaluated. An aim of asthma therapy is to use the optimum medication needed to maintain control of the disease with minimal risk.

The step-care approach to treatment, in which the number of medications and their frequency of use are increased only as necessary, is helpful.

Continual monitoring—with pulmonary function tests and reevaluation of the benefits of medication, as well as an awareness of the allergic triggers and what is being done to avoid them— is a necessary component of any treatment plan for the asthmatic.

In order to attain these goals, patient education, environmental measures, pulmonary function tests and proper administration of medications are an absolute necessity. At the present time there is no expectation the disease can be cured.

Despite the fact this cannot be cured, there are several world class athletes with asthma, including Jackie Joyner-Kersee, considered by some to be the greatest woman athlete of the twentieth century, who won Olympic gold in the heptathalon and the long jump in 1988 and was diagnosed with asthma in 1982. Several swimmers qualified in preliminary trials for the Atlanta Olympics 1996. These superb athletes, whose well-publicized control of their asthma and their continued ability to perform despite the disease, have given national attention to asthma, and their accomplishments have given hope to countless sufferers.

Los Angeles asthma and allergy specialist Roger Katz, who has many elite athletes as patients, says that the so-called stop-and-go sports, such as wrestling, weight training, softball, doubles tennis and swimming are excellent choices for people with asthma. He hopes to be able to highlight and publicize the careers of successful athletes who have worked out a plan of effective management with an asthma specialist to demonstrate that it is possible to play and compete successfully at demanding sports, as well as live a full and complete life with the condition.

Diagnosis

The diagnosis of asthma should be considered for anyone who wheezes. Asthma is the most likely diagnosis when wheezing starts in childhood or early adulthood, and is interspersed with periods without any symptoms.

It is estimated that over ninety percent of all asthmatics lack adequate medical help. Many doctors and patients underestimate the seriousness of asthma, causing it to go under-treated, and causing asthmatics to suffer needless anxiety, discomfort and, sometimes, death. A campaign by the National Asthma Education Program, led by Albert L. Sheffer, hopes to change the lives of millions by providing a comprehensive outline of the causes of asthma and its diagnosis and treatment. The goal of the campaign is to provide patients with more effective treatment, and to encourage asthmatics to monitor their breathing capacity with a device that can warn of attacks in time to prevent their occurrence.

Black children suffer from asthma more than their white counterparts. Dr. Floyd Malveaux, chairman of the Department of Microbiology at Howard University's Department of Medicine, says that the death rates from asthma are also higher in black children than in white children.

Under examination, blood and sputum will usually show eosinophilia (white blood cells). The sputum is highly distinctive. It is tenacious, rubbery and whitish. With an infection, particularly in adults, the sputum may be yellowish.

Chest x-rays may not be the best diagnostic tool, as the findings may vary on the same individuals during their lifetime, depending upon their activity and life-style.

Pulmonary function tests are useful in known asthmatics for assessing the degree of airways obstruction, and measuring airway response to inhaled allergens and chemicals. Testing is most valuable diagnostically when performed before and after using an aerosol bronchodilator to determine the degree of reversibility of airway obstruction.

Static lung volumes and capacities can reveal various combinations of abnormalities. However no abnormalities may be detected when most cases are in remission.

Dynamic lung volumes and capacities provide an index of airway obstruction. These are reduced in asthmatics and return to normal following administration of an aerosolized bronchodilator.

The assessment of other factors is more difficult. Nonspecific irritants (particularly cigarette smoke) and evidence of infection (usually viral) should always be evaluated.

Attacks related to environmental allergen exposures, or a history of rhinitis (inflammation of the mucous membrane of the nose) suggest the likelihood of outside allergic factors.

Confirming such allergies is best accomplished by an allergy evaluation that includes allergy skin testing to detect common inhalants (pollens, molds, skin scales of furred animals, house dust mites) suggested by the history of the patient.

Exercise testing using a treadmill or bicycle ergometer has been found to be useful, particularly in children, to confirm undecided diagnoses. Over 90% of children with asthma will develop a post exercise fall in pulmonary function.

The National Institutes of Health classifies asthma based on the response to medication as follows:

Mild asthma—mild and episodic that requires inhaled beta-agonists less than 2 times per week.

Moderate asthma—not controlled with as-needed use of inhaled beta-agonists. The addition of inhaled corticosteroids, sustained-release theophyllines, or oral beta-agonists is required.

Severe asthma—not controlled on maximum doses of bronchodilators (oral and inhaled) and an inhaled anti-inflammatory agent.

Treatment

The first step in any treatment of asthma, after diagnosis, is to focus on preventing or reversing the airway inflammation that is the main cause of the hypersensitive response of the airway.

Each individual asthmatic differs in the therapy required. The severity of the condition, the tolerance to medication and sensitivity to environmental allergens must be considered.

The role of environmental factors should be rigorously investigated. If suspected, allergy skin tests should confirm the history.

Individual triggers must be reduced, avoided or eliminated. Known allergens and irritants should be recognized—such as animal dander, carpets, dust, and molds—and these should be eliminated from the environment as much as possible. A living environment tailored to the needs of the individual should be possible without too much disruption of the lives of the rest of the family.

In the bedroom the focus should be to eliminate as many irritants as possible, as this is where you spend approximately one-third of your time.

Mattress and box springs should be placed in an impermeable zippered casing, and carpeting should be removed, particularly in a warm, moist climate that favors the growth of mildew.

Other allergens (dust mites, mold and pollens) may be selected for a trial of allergy immuno-therapy (formerly termed hyposensitization). Improvement should be noted within 12 to 24 months after beginning treatment. If no significant improvement is noted within this time, immunotherapy should be stopped. When improvement occurs, the optimum duration of therapy is unknown but at least three years is recommended.

Nonspecific factors which make the condition worse (e.g., cigarette smoke, odors, irritant fumes, changes in temperature, atmospheric pressure, and humidity) should be investigated and controlled if possible.

Aspirin should be avoided, particularly in those with nasal polyps, because of aspirin-induced asthma.

Sensitivity to sulfites (used widely as food preservatives) is suggested when attacks follow eating from a salad bar or drinking red wine or beer.

The *Self Care Catalogue* (1-800-345-3371) and *Allergy Free Inc.* (1-800-Allergy) both list a number of products which may be beneficial, such as:

> an ultra-hygienic pillow and other anti-allergy bedding that is dust mite proof;

> a fabric spray that keeps dust mite allergens out of the air;
>
> a nonirritating spray that prevents pet dander from becoming airborne;
>
> a dry mop that uses disposable polyethylene-fiber dusting sheets that attract and hold dust with a static charge;
>
> electrostatic air cleaners, air filters and vacuum cleaners;
>
> and even washable stuffed animals made with no plastic parts.

In addition, there are a variety of home air purifiers which recycle bedroom or living space air and remove airborne irritants down to 0.3 microns. These can be purchased from air conditioner manufacturers, hardware stores, retail outlets, and a variety of other sources.

British researchers, reporting in *The Lancet* in 1996, reported that women who cook on gas stoves are at greater risk of asthma attacks and other respiratory symptoms than women who use other cooking methods.

High concentrations of nitrogen dioxide, a product of natural gas which can adversely affect the lungs, may be the cause. In this new study of over 1,000 British adults, women who said they cooked with gas were more likely to have experienced wheezing, breathlessness, asthma attacks and hay fever during the previous year than those who did not cook with gas.

Lead researcher Deborah Jarvis, of St. Thomas' Hospital in London, theorized that the women exposed themselves to levels of gas that were higher in the kitchen than elsewhere in the home. Based on this study, the authors estimated that asthma attacks in women could be reduced up to sixty-seven percent if they stopped using gas stoves, while wheezing could be reduced by eleven to thirty-nine percent.

This association is not entirely new, according to R. Michael Sly, chief of allergy and immunology at the Children's National Medical Center in Washington D.C. He stated that adverse effects have long been reported from wood-burning stoves or passive smoking. In each case, there is a different specific mechanism, but they all seem to increase airway irritation.

Researchers stress that gas cooking could have important public-health consequences. As many as sixty percent of people in most European and North American countries use gas appliances, and that exposure is common, and possibly increasing, throughout the world.

Dr. Sly suggests that anyone with respiratory conditions use other means of cooking, such as electricity, whenever possible.

According to Australian researchers, a diet high in sugar and fat may be a contributing factor in the development of asthma among children with common allergies. Thus, promoting a healthy diet can prevent the development of asthma symptoms, according to Jennifer K. Peat, MD, a senior research officer in the department of medicine at the University of Sydney. The researchers recorded the dietary habits of children susceptible to common allergies. They also measured the children's abilities to breathe normally while exercising. The children who showed signs of airway hyper-responsiveness ate twenty-three percent more refined sugar and twenty-five percent more high-fat foods than those who did not.

Others have suggested that excess weight was obstructing lung function in the children with airway hyper-responsiveness.

The Australian dietary study also confirmed that children with a higher intake of fish oil appear to have fewer symptoms of asthma. This research links diet to asthma, and is similar to research of fifteen years earlier that linked saturated fats and heart disease. As yet there is not a firm association, but Mike White, spokesperson for the American Thoracic Society, states that evidence is evolving in that direction.

There are five groups of drugs that are useful in the treatment and control of asthma.

1. B-Adrenergic agents

   These drugs cause bronchial smooth muscle relaxation and may inhibit small vascular leakage into the airway. They include epinephrine, isoproterenol and some more selective B2-adrenergics. The B2-adrenergics have more bronchodilatory effects and less cardiostimulatory effect. The commonly used B2s include metaproterenol, terbutaline, isoetharine, albuterol, bitolterol, and pibuterol.

   In general, epinephrine by injection and one of the B2 agents inhaled are most useful in treating an acute attack. After inhalation, the B2s have a rapid onset of action (within minutes) but are active for only four to six hours at most. B2s are the drugs of choice to relieve acute asthma attacks and to prevent broncho-constriction following exercise or other stimulation. Adverse effects are dose-related: they are more common after oral than aerosol administration because of the much higher dose required for oral drugs. Sustained-release medications help prevent nocturnal asthma.

2. Theophylline (a methylxanthine) relaxes bronchial smooth muscle. Its mechanism decreases small vascular leakage, inhibits the late response to allergens, and may inhibit other chemical mediators.

   Theophylline is a valuable companion to the adrenergic drugs for management of acute episodes, particularly in those who do not respond to the highest aerosol bronchodilator therapy. Oral theophylline is very useful in the management of nocturnal asthma.

3. Oral and intravenous corticosteroids

   Corticosteroids inhibit the attraction of leukocytes to the site of an allergic reaction and stimulate B2 receptors. They block the late response to inhaled allergens and the subsequent bronchial hyper-responsiveness it causes. With long-term therapy, bronchial hyper-responsiveness gradually decreases. While corticosteroids given intravenously are particularly effective, they are reserved for more difficult episodes because of their potential for adverse effects. Short-term use in high dosage (five to seven days to abort an attack) is not usually associated with significant harmful side effects. The new surface-active inhaled steroids are useful for maintenance therapy, but not for managing acute episodes.

Oral or intravenous corticosteroids, such as prednisone, prednisolone or medrol are often used in the early treatment of severe acute asthma attacks to prevent their progression and reduce the severity of the disease. These medications, taken orally, can often reduce the need for trips to the emergency room and subsequent hospitalization. Their action occurs approximately three hours after they are taken, and they peak at six to twelve hours.

However, corticoid steroids, which are hormones, have many adverse effects.

Short-term major adverse effects include reversible abnormalities in sugar metabolism, increased appetite, mood alteration, high blood pressure, and stomach or duodenal ulcers.

Long-term risks include osteoporosis, hypertension, cataracts, and impaired functioning of the immune system.

4. Inhaled corticosteroids

    Inhaled corticosteroids are relatively safe and are used as primary therapy for moderate and severe asthma. They provide symptomatic relief and reduce the hyper-responsiveness of the airway.

5. Croolyn sodium

    This medication is given preventively. It inhibits allergen-induced airway narrowing. It also inhibits acute airway hyper-activity after exercise or exposure to cold dry air. It is sometimes necessary to have a four to six week trial therapy to determine if you will respond. It is primarily useful for children and some adults for maintenance therapy only. While problems with patient compliance appear to have limited its use, it is the safest of all drugs used to treat asthma.

6. Anticholinergic agents

    Atropine and ipratropium bromide block certain pathways that cause airways obstruction. They may provide added bronchodilator effects in those already receiving inhaled B2-agents.

7. Bronchodilators

They dilate the airways by relaxing bronchial smooth muscle. They include beta-adrenergic agonists, methylxanthines, and anticholinergics.

Inhaled beta-adrenergic agonists are the medication of choice for treatment of acute increases in the severity of asthma and for the prevention of exercise-induced asthma. In addition, they are used in the control of persistent airway narrowing. The latest research, however, suggests prolonged, regular administration (as opposed to as-necessary use) of a potent inhaled beta-agonist might result in diminished control of asthma and in some cases it has been suggested they have been a contributing factor in asthmatic death. The well-publicized death of the teenage Krissy Taylor, sister of model Nikki Taylor, in 1995 brought media attention to the consequences of the overuse of such an inhalant. These agonists should only be used for acute airway obstruction. They are best administered via metered dose inhaler or nebulizer.

The drug theophylline is the principal methylxanthine used in asthma therapy for relaxation and dilation of the bronchi. When used in a sustained release form, it has a long duration of action and is particularly useful in the control of nighttime asthma. However, it has the potential for significant adverse effects if used excessively. Nausea and vomiting are the earliest signs of toxicity, continuing on to a rapid heart rate, abnormal heart rhythms, as well as elevated blood sugar and potassium levels. It is best that theophylline blood levels are monitored when beginning therapy and at regular intervals of six to twelve months thereafter. Aminophylline, another methylxanthine, is also available by rectal suppository.

Anticholinergics are infrequently used because of the length of time they take to act and because of a number of unpleasant side effects.

Over-the-counter bronchodilators are available. Some of them contain both theophylline and ephedrine (adrenaline) and act as decongestants also. Because some people think over-the-counter medications are not as strong as prescription medications, there is a temptation to think dosages can be increased without harm. This is not true. These are powerful drugs and should be only taken for acute attacks—not on a regular basis. The dosage outlined should be adhered to religiously, and the doctor supervising the asthmatic should be aware that these over-the-counter medications have been taken.

8. Expectorants

Because there is a quantity of thick mucus in the airways of the asthmatic, it is helpful to take an expectorant in conjunction with a bronchodilator. Expectorants thin the mucus and make it easier to cough it up. Because ridding the airways of this thick mucus is helpful, a cough suppressant is not recommended. Prescription expectorants contain either guaifenesin or iodinated glycerol.

Most over-the counter expectorants contain only guaifenesin.

Several combination prescription drugs contain both a bronchodilator and an expectorant, and are available in tablets and liquid.

Over-the-counter combinations contain theophylline, ephedrine and guaifenesin, and several others contain these same three ingredients plus Phenobarbital.

Because of the variety of combinations, it is best to have the recommendation of your physician before you purchase any over-the-counter medication for the temporary relief of acute attacks.

9. Peak-flow meters

Just as a diabetic measures blood-sugar, an asthmatic should have a peak-flow meter to measure breathing ability. This device should be used daily to measure the maximum air speed of exhaling a deep breath; by comparing that value with their personal best, asthma patients can adjust their bronchodilator medication as needed to relieve or even avoid symptoms.

Any asthmatic who does not have a peak-
flow meter to use daily should request
one from the doctor.

Asthma is classified by its response to drug therapy
and how these drugs allow you to manage your
condition.

Since it is well known that asthma worsens at
night, tightening airways as the person sleeps, new
research suggests that medicine is needed before
the airways begin to tighten in the early morning
hours. Dosing for optimal benefit will help to keep
the airways open at night. "Dosing at 3 PM is much
better than at the traditional 8 in the morning or
8 in the evening," says Dr. Richard J. Martin, MD,
Professor of Medicine, University of Colorado Health
Sciences Center. "If you use an inhaler with steroid medicine, it is a good idea to take one of
those doses between 3 and 5 PM to obtain peak
effect overnight."

However, the asthmatic needs to take an active role in managing the disease, in the planning
of activities and the avoidance of triggers, rather
than relying solely on medication to control attacks when they occur.

Often, the asthmatic who takes an active role
in planning and avoiding triggers can lead a far
more satisfactory and normal life, despite the

severity of the condition, than those who simply rely on medication to treat the symptoms.

Treating Allergy

The immune response is a measure the body takes to protect itself from a foreign substance. However, immune responses can become exaggerated and lead to various types of tissue damage.

Hypersensitivity or allergy is an inappropriate and abnormal response to antigens originating outside the body. The allergic state results in asthma, hay fever and allergies—to food, drugs, plants and other environmental factors.

Whereas the immune response is a protective adaptive response designed to guard the body against the invasion of dangerous toxic substances, the allergic response is an oversensitive and often harmful response on the part of the body against foreign substances that may actually be harmless, e.g. plant pollens.

In other words, in the immune response the body's protective cells correctly recognize dangerous intruders, fight them, and often destroy them. Conversely, in allergic response the body's protective cells overestimate the danger from a harmless intruder, start a battle and in the end, produce needless damage to the body's tissues.

The word "allergy" (from *allos*, other and *ergon*, energy) signifies that the activity or energy of the body has in some way been altered.

An allergy is a response, unique to that individual, that develops as a result of exposure to a pollen, food, dust, plant or animals. Such allergies are widespread in the general population and it is not unusual to hear many complaints about the pollen count or particular foods or medications because allergies are so commonplace.

This hypersensitivity is an abnormal or unusual reaction to an agent (usually a protein) that does not normally produce symptoms in most people. Thus, only certain people are allergic to pollens, while certain other people are allergic to strawberries.

An allergen can be defined as any substance with the capacity to create a hypersensitive state or an allergy within the body. Although allergens are highly variable in their chemical makeup, most are protein in nature, with a few exceptions, such as plant oils.

The major types of allergens are categorized as inhalants, ingestants, contactants, injectants, and infectants.

In interesting early research, Steven L. Kagen, assistant clinical professor of allergy and immunology at the Medical College of Wisconsin, Appleton, states that Helicobacter pylori, a bacteria in the stomach, may cause allergies. This theory, presented at the American Academy of Allergy and Immunology, marks the first time that scientists have suggested that it is possible to be allergic to bacteria. Dr. Kagen states that this finding could help people with allergies be properly diagnosed. He adds that if future studies back his findings, allergy symptoms could be alleviated merely by getting the H. pylori bacteria out of the stomach, usually with a course of antibiotics.

Eric Ottesen, a parasitologist and allergist who heads the Clinical Parasitology Section at the National Institute of Allergy and Infectious Diseases, thinks that allergies may be the result of a misdirected effort by the body to rid itself of parasitic worms. Parasitic worms, including filarial worms, hookworms, whipworms, pinworms, and flatworms, affect more than two billion people throughout the world, causing afflictions from elephantiasis to blindness to serious intestinal problems. Ottesen made the connection between parasites and allergy on a research trip to the South Pacific island of Mauke. Nineteen years after he began treating islanders for parasites, Ottesen found that parasitic infections were down, but there was much more allergy. Similar findings elsewhere in the world have convinced him that there is a link. He believes that when the immune system is no longer fighting parasites, it seeks new targets, such as allergens. At the moment, this is an interesting but unsubstantiated theory.

Inhalants include plant pollens and dusts. They may create such problems as seasonal hay fever, seasonal asthma and allergic rhinitis. Tissues that are particularly vulnerable to inhalants are the mucosa of the eye, nose and the bronchi.

Ingestants include foods and drugs. Allergies to ingestants may manifest themselves as rhinitis, asthma, diarrhea, colitis, abdominal pain, dermatitis, itching skin and migraine headaches. The major organs and tissues affected by ingestants are the mucosa of the nose and the bronchi, the gastrointestinal tract, the skin and the brain.

Contactants include soaps and plants, and mainly affect the skin, resulting in such problems as contact dermatitis.

Injectants include such preparations as foreign sera (liquids) or drugs; these substances can affect any tissue in the body, causing drug allergy and serum sickness.

Infectants or bacteria can also infect any tissue in the body.

The final group of allergens are termed autoallergens. They are altered and modified tissue allergens that have become so changed by physical, chemical or infective agents they can cause a hypersensitive reaction within the individual. The allergens, then, develop within the body rather than entering as a foreign substance from the outside environment. These allergens play an important role in the cause of autoimmune disease.

The precise factors causing allergy are not known; however, heredity, congenital factors and contact between an individual and an allergen are known to play important roles in the development of allergic reactions.

First of all, heredity has been linked with the beginning of allergies because some allergies definitely appear to run in families. Also, allergies appear to affect one tenth of the population more frequently and more severely than other individuals within the population. Heredity evidently not only determines that a particular individual will be allergic, but also determines the type of allergy that person will experience, as well as the precise allergens to which he will be susceptible.

Congenital factors can influence an individual's susceptibility to allergens, because allergens can definitely be passed to the fetus via placental circulation. Such an allergic sensitivity is not the result of heredity, but is acquired: the fetus is actively sensitized during prenatal life. For example, if a mother, during pregnancy, eats large amounts of a particular food, the child may become overly sensitized to that particular protein while still within the mother's womb. After birth, when the child comes into contact with that food, she may then manifest certain signs of allergy.

A final important factor in allergy is contact between the person and a particular allergen. Although heredity plays a role in predisposing an individual to the development of a particular allergy, heredity alone cannot cause a person to become allergic. Contact with an allergen is essential to the development of any allergy. On the other hand, in certain allergies such as seasonal hay fever and allergic asthma, contact with the allergen is not sufficient in itself to produce the allergy, because heredity is a major factor. For example, although thousands of people within our population are exposed to certain seasonal pollens every year, only a limited number of persons, with a certain hereditary predisposition toward allergic reactions, develop seasonal hay fever.

There are certain precipitating or modifying factors that also influence the development of allergies. The most important are stress, infection, endocrine disturbances and in some cases, pregnancy. Such factors can upset the balance between allergenic surroundings and the individual with a hereditary predisposition toward development of allergy. For example, some pregnant women experience severe bronchial asthma attacks for the first time in their lives. Similarly, certain individuals, when under great stress, will break out in hives. Thus, the mental state of an individual and his physical state both profoundly influence whether the individual with a hereditary predisposition toward allergy will actually develop an allergy.

The treatment of allergies or hay fever includes removing yourself from exposure to the offending allergen, medication and sometimes desensitization injections.

Michael Kaliner, the head of allergic diseases at the National Institutes of Health, says all the bad allergens in the United States can be found in Washington, D.C., but Washington is nevertheless not the worst city for allergy sufferers; based on this observation he believes it is not worthwhile to try to avoid allergies by moving.

As an example of how futile it is to move to avoid known allergens, University of Southern California researcher Kathleen Rodgers and colleague Dolph Ellefson found low doses of the insecticide Malathion caused an allergic rash and allergy symptoms following aerial spraying there to destroy fruit flies. She found the Malathion acted directly on the immune cells to release histamine, which triggered allergy symptoms, causing a new set of problems for individuals who had not been allergic prior to the spraying of the pesticide. There are always new things introduced into any environment, so avoiding millions of possible allergens by moving is hardly feasible.

Since the majority of known causative agents include cigarette smoke, pollen, dust, dander, foods and chemicals, it is easy to see that identifying the agent or agents can be complex. Avoiding exposure can be difficult. However, it is possible to be aware of immediate reactions to things such as cigarette smoke or pet dander. When the allergen is more difficult to identify (and it is seldom there is just one), skin testing can often be used to isolate and identify the offending agent. Then it is possible to become aware of exposure and take steps to lessen that exposure.

One area seldom considered when individuals try removing the offending allergen is the family automobile. The upholstery should be thoroughly washed, particularly if the family pet is often taken along when traveling.

It is also important allergies not be mistaken for colds because the symptoms are so similar. A proper diagnosis from an allergist is crucial to begin the process of relieving allergy symptoms.

Some of the steps taken by an asthmatic may also make life easier for the allergic individual.

Pollen exposure can be limited by staying indoors in air-conditioning during the worst of the season.

The National Institutes of Health recommend removing carpeting, upholstered furniture, heavy curtains or drapes, venetian blinds, fuzzy wool blankets and comforters stuffed with wool or down feathers. They suggest the bedroom, in particular, be scrubbed down, as well as all the furniture, which would be best to be plastic or metal that can be washed, and it be thoroughly cleaned weekly. Clothing should be kept in plastic zippered bags, and shoes in closed boxes off the floor.

According to Australian researchers, individuals who carefully launder bed linens and avoid rugs and stuffed animals to protect themselves from dust mites should turn their attention to their own clothing.

In a study conducted at the University of Sydney, researchers tested the clothing of twenty university workers, collecting dust samples with a small, portable vacuum cleaner.

More than half of the garments had allergen levels that would provoke a reaction in people sensitive to dust mites, and ten percent had levels high enough to induce an asthma attack.

Mites burrow into clothing because perspiration provides a moist environment, and they can feed on shed skin cells, according to Thomas Platts-Mills of the University of Virginia in Charlottesville.

The solution is as close and as cheap as the washing machine, according to the Australian researchers. Washing clothing in hot water—at least 131°F—kills most bugs; cold water removes more than ninety-five percent of the dust-mite debris, but significant numbers of mites can survive the cold water. Although cold water washing might protect the colors in washable clothing, it is not worth the savings in the life of garments for allergic individuals.

Allergy sufferers should look for fabrics that stand up to regular washing and hot temperatures, and avoid clothing that must be dry-cleaned, because most people tend to have these items cleaned less often than washable clothing.

A new generation of anti-allergen vacuum cleaners is now available that can capture allergy-inducing particles that conventional vacuums miss. Conventional vacuums merely pull in dust and deposit it in a porous bag. Anti-allergy vacuums, however, draw incoming air through a series of increasingly fine filters that prevent almost all particles from escaping.

Consumer Reports on Health in May, 1996 suggest that pollen exposure can be minimized by keeping doors and windows shut, changing the filter on the air conditioner frequently, and avoiding yard work that stirs up pollen. If you must cut the grass or rake leaves, cover both your eyes and nose with goggles and a dust mask (sold in hardware stores everywhere); minimize outdoor activity before 10 AM. when the pollen counts are usually highest; if you exercise outdoors, wait until the evening when the pollen count will be lower.

Avoiding allergenic foods can be relatively simple, once they are recognized. Read labels when food shopping, and ask about the ingredients of various dishes when eating out.

Avoidance of animals who cause allergic reactions is slightly more difficult, but there are some pets that create fewer difficulties than others, such as fish.

A major allergen in the pet dander classification is cat dander. However, it is possible to have a cat in the home and avoid the allergic response with a small amount of extra effort. Cat allergens are a result of the natural and regular shedding of tiny flakes of skin. These flakes are mixed with shed fur and the cat's saliva which contains a protein called Fel D1. This mix of skin, fur and saliva (dander) becomes airborne when the animal scratches. It can rub off onto your skin and clothing when the pet is held or stroked, or when you sit on furniture where the cat has been. Washing the cat once a month in lukewarm distilled water will cause the cat to stop making this allergen after approximately three to eight months. This washing neither harms the cat nor removes too much oil from its fur. A variety of cat care books can provide suggestions on teaching the cat to tolerate bathing, such as placing a towel on the bottom of the sink so that the cat can have something non-slippery under its feet.

One unusual allergy is an allergy to sex. Some women find they are allergic to their partner's semen, and other people find any sort of physical exertion leads to the sneezes and allergic reactions. Latex condoms are the most common cause of sexual allergies, however. Allergy medication and desensitization regimens can help, and condom users should consider wearing a natural membrane condom over or under the latex condom, depending on which partner needs the shielding.

It is the responsibility of the allergic individual to be alert to offending allergens and to avoid them as quickly as possible. Research suggests that the symptoms of allergies, such as sneezing, red itching eyes, wheezing and coughing, usually are the worst in the morning and that timing antihistamine and anti-inflammatories to the symptoms may block them before they peak. A large study in France showed that antihistamines were most effective when most or all of the daily dose was taken at dinner time.

According to the French researchers, each individual should observe when they have peak symptoms and keep a record of them in a small notebook. Once you have determined when your symptoms are appearing, you can then determine when is the best time to take your medicine to ward off an allergy attack.

According to allergist Romi Saini, of the Johns Hopkins Asthma and Allergy Center in Baltimore, new treatments include prescription inhalers, most of which are low-dose steroid nasal sprays that can head off an allergic reaction before it starts.

For temporary relief of mild allergies, in addition to avoiding the triggers, antihistamines are the most commonly used medication.

Prescription options now include several which are non-sedating.

A number of over-the-counter antihistamines are available and they are either alone or in combination with decongestants. If the allergies are mild, it is possible to try an over-the-counter product before moving on to a prescription one, as a less expensive option.

Antihistamine eye drops can be beneficial if tearing is a problem.

Nasal irrigation will enhance the action of any

of the anti-allergy medications as it will remove mucus secretions as well as pollen and dust.

If allergies are seasonal, it is wise to be aware of that, and avoid as many outdoor activities as possible during the active pollen season.

If the symptomatic relief provided by avoidance of the allergen is insufficient, if antihistamines and nasal sprays are inadequate to control the condition, it is suggested you see an allergist.

After a battery of skin tests, in which minute particles of well-known allergens are inserted under the skin to look for a reaction, allergy desensitization injections might be recommended.

A study reported in the *New England Journal of Medicine* may aid in resolving the seventy-year old debate about the use of allergy shots to treat allergic asthma. This study, published in February of 1996, showed the shots may help asthmatics to breathe easier and use other medications less. About thirty percent of adults with asthma have this form of asthma which is triggered or worsened by certain materials, such as pollen.

However, this same study also showed that the injections may not work for everyone and may have only a limited effect on symptoms. For those who have tried other asthma treatments without success or experienced side effects, hyposensitization injections might be something to consider.

These injections will slowly increase your body's tolerance to the offending substance. It has been found that these injections appear to benefit those allergic to pollens far more than those allergic to mold, dust-mites and animal danders.

Treating Bronchitis

Acute Bronchitis

Acute bronchitis may develop after a common cold or other viral infection. It is generally self-limiting with eventual complete healing.

Rest is indicated until the fever subsides. An increase in oral fluids and an analgesic such as acetaminophen taken every four to six hours will reduce the fever and aid in treating the general bodily discomfort.

Chronic Bronchitis

Chronic bronchitis is associated with prolonged exposure to bronchial irritants. As a result of that exposure, there is mucus hypersecretion and certain bronchi structural changes. The most observable characteristic is a chronic productive cough.

Any treatment of chronic bronchitis is aimed at opening the airways and improving the symptomatic signs (wheezing, coughing, viscid sputum) of the illness. If a person with chronic bronchitis continues to smoke cigarettes, it will not be possible to present any kind of effective program.

IF YOU ARE SMOKING, YOU MUST GET HELP TO STOP. IMMEDIATELY.

There can be no clearer statement that can be made than to say:

THE WORST THING YOU CAN DO FOR YOUR CONDITION IS TO CONTINUE USING CIGARETTES.

After the cessation of smoking, the physician can prescribe a combination of drugs, depending on the severity of the condition and whether or not there is infection present.

An expectorant will aid in loosening the mucus by decreasing its thickness. When the mucus is thinned, the cilia will be able to do their work in moving the accumulated secretions up and out of the lungs and bronchial tubes.

A cough suppressant is *not* recommended as it will stop the coughing and prevent the removal of this infected mucus.

Eight glasses of water daily will aid in thinning the secretions; inhaling highly polluted, cold or dry air should be avoided.

Chronic bronchitis is just that, a chronic condition. It requires consistent and persistent treatment. If chronic bronchitis is allowed to continue for any length of time, the bronchial walls will eventually thicken and the number of mucous glands will increase, adding to the discomfort and the possibility of further disease, sometimes becoming chronic obstructive bronchitis.

Anyone with chronic bronchitis who has a cold or influenza should be given an antibiotic to prevent a secondary infection, such as acute bronchitis or pneumonia. Both these conditions are caused by bacteria, but pneumonia is the most severe and serious of the two infections.

Sinobronchitis

Frequently acute sinusitis and acute bronchitis can be present in one individual at the same time. All the symptoms of sinusitis will be present, along with a persistent deep, wet-sounding cough which will be productive of a yellow-green mucus. The person suffering both of these conditions at the same time will frequently feel quite ill and feverish, with little appetite, and with a great deal of fatigue, as the difficulty in breathing and the constant coughing often prevent restful sleep. Both these conditions are treated with antibiotics; the objective is to open and drain the obstructed sinus cavity of its infected mucus, and to remove the infected mucus from the bronchi of the lungs.

Steam, whether from the shower or from a humidifier, is beneficial for both conditions as it will loosen and thin the secretions from both the sinuses and the bronchi.

After steaming, postural drainage (described below) is an excellent treatment for the mucus in the airway. It clears the lungs of retained and infected secretions by using gravity to move the material instead of relying on the normal bronchial clearing mechanisms (which may be impaired as the result of disease). A controlled study by Lorin and Denning demonstrated that postural drainage produced more than twice the amount of sputum produced by an equal period of coughing without it. Postural draining not only rids the lungs of infected material, it also minimizes coughing. Postural drainage is best performed by having another person cup their hands and clap lightly and rhythmically on both the back and then the chest of the patient as he is either seated in a chair and leaning forward or lying head down. (Cupping the hands makes the impact on the body air-cushioned for a short period of time.) This can aid in drainage of mucus, which then can be more easily coughed up. Several pillows placed on a bed, just under the lower part of the abdomen will allow the upper part of the body to relax forward on the bed, or lying head down on a slant board (an ironing board will do). This position will allow gravity to assist in draining the mucus from the lungs. Clapping should begin about mid back and work upward toward the shoulders, including the shoulder blades, and then in front from the lower ribs up to the collar bone. For the female, the breasts should be avoided but clapping can be performed on the area above the breasts up to the collar bone. This process should take about twenty minutes and should never be done forcefully or hard enough to injure, or cause pain or discomfort. A light touch is sufficient to assist in dislodging the mucus.

It is possible to perform a similar action on yourself by rhythmically tapping with your fingertips on your chest. These movements, made with the fingertips of both hands, cause vibrations in the chest that will help to dislodge secretions.

Your physician, a nurse or a respiratory therapist can demonstrate these techniques to you or other family members who will assist you in postural drainage.

Chronic Obstructive Bronchitis

Chronic obstructive bronchitis is a disease of the small airways, of a sufficient degree to lead to a significant airways obstruction. It is the result of prolonged exposure to bronchial irritants.

Treatment may slow the progression of the disorder and may consist of:

A broad-spectrum antibiotic.

Systemic hydration.

Mist inhalation, postural drainage and chest physical therapy.

Avoidance of bronchial irritants (especially smoking).

A diagnosis of chronic disease should be taken seriously, as anyone with untreated disease will become increasingly susceptible to lung infections such as acute bronchitis and pneumonia, which can ultimately lead to emphysema.

Chronic lung disease, consisting primarily of bronchitis and emphysema, is currently the fourth leading cause of death for Americans.

Section IV

Are You Ready for Healthy Sinuses?

You have had a number of sinus infections, and every time you get sick you always end up with a sinus condition. When you get a cold, you dread what is to follow, because you know it will be sinusitis.

You get a number of upper respiratory infections each year, ending in sinusitis—you take a course of antibiotics and then you are better for a while. But ...finally when the antibiotics are done, you find yourself right back where you started and you are sick and tired of it—and so are your poor aching sinuses.

Pain, fever and fatigue are all messages from your body. It is time to listen to it; it is asking you to help it get well, to make the changes necessary for health.

It is no longer enough to treat the sinus infection after you have it; you want to avoid getting this infection in the first place. Reestablishing immune system defenses is an essential part in overcoming repeated sinuses infections.

Are you are ready to take charge of your sinus health?

If you have an active sinus infection, you must take a prescribed course of antibiotics in order to permit the damaged mucous membranes of the nose and sinuses to properly heal.

The sinus cavities in the head communicate with veins that drain from the brain. Brain abscesses, meningitis, or cavernous sinus thrombosis in the brain are all rare but real potential complications of sinusitis. For that reason, as well as the possibility of permanent damage to the sinus membranes, you cannot permit a sinus infection to persist indefinitely.

As all infections, when your health is continually being undermined, when all the other measures you have taken do not work within a reasonable period of time, or the severity of the condition dictates it, antibiotics must be used.

However, if you have decided to improve your own health, if you have decided that you do not want to learn to live with this condition and the diminished quality of life it provides, then it is time to take a look at all things you have to do to take charge and change your life.

If you have decided you would rather change your life than go for that quick fix; if you would rather stop focusing on your sinusitis and then just treating the symptoms when you suffer from them, then you are ready to do what is necessary to become truly healthy with healthy sinuses.

The Inner Environment—Building an Optimum Immune System

A strong and healthy immune system will defend the body against invading pathogens. When viruses or bacteria attack, your immune system springs into action. That defensive response involves the effort from phagocytes, macrophages, antibodies and lymphocytes: all cells whose job it is to attack and destroy these invaders.

In order to sustain such a defense, a whole bevy of nutrients and other factors are required to forge the components of these phagocytes, macrophages, antibodies and lymphocytes; to sustain their efforts and to replenish your store of them when the battle is over, in preparation for the next onslaught. Your body's resources for doing this are not unlimited. It takes a complete storehouse of factors to keep your immune system healthy and operating at full capacity.

You need stress control, rest, sleep, a healthy diet, and proper hygiene for your immune system to operate at its optimum capacity.

Before you say, "Oh, no, I'm not interested in reading that I have to make some elaborate change in life-style!" read on. It might be that some simple part of these suggestions might make all the difference in your condition. Also, if you do make life-style changes, you just might find that you feel so much better that it will be well worth it.

Hygiene

Viruses are everywhere. They are on almost every surface and live on our skin without harm to us most of the time.

The greatest single thing anyone can do to prevent transmission of viruses, not only into our own respiratory tract but to others, is thorough hand washing. When we accept change for a purchase from a clerk in a store, take a file folder from another individual in the office, use the telephone right after someone with a cold, we are at risk. As the world gets smaller, as people travel all over the globe, it provides the opportunity for a great variety of new viruses to travel great distances, exposing us to many we might never have met a decade or so ago.

Paranoia about the prevalence of viruses is not the answer. Avoiding friends, refusing to hug our children or wearing a surgical mask will not do much to prevent the spread of viruses either.

Routine hygiene: bathing, keeping the kitchen and the house clean, careful washing of eating utensils, dishes, glasses; not sharing lipsticks or sipping from another person's drink—these are standard things that we all think everyone takes for granted. They should be considered routine preventive hygiene.

However, most of us are unaware of how many times a day we touch our faces, our noses, our lips and our eyes with our fingers. We push hair off of our faces, we scratch our noses, we take finger foods into our mouths, we pull our lashes to get something out of our eyes; many of us touch our faces hundreds of times a day without even being aware of it. Because we touch many things that have been touched by others during the course of daily living, we are bound to come in contact with a lot of different pathogens. Most of them never harm us, and our immune system goes right to work creating a defense against any invasion.

Our own hands are one of the greatest sources of transmission of viruses into our system. Thorough hand washing is one of the most simple and beneficial things we can do for ourselves to prevent the spread of viruses.

When you do have a cold or the flu, sneeze into a disposable tissue instead of your hands, and if you do sneeze into your hands, wash them so you don't re-infect yourself. Teach your children to sneeze into their own shoulder by turning their head to the side when they feel a sneeze coming on, rather than into their hands or directly into the room as children seldom carry tissues or have them handy.

Alcohol-Nicotine-Caffeine

Decrease alcohol intake. Alcohol not only adds non-nutritious calories, it contributes to depression, fatigue and anxiety. It lowers inhibitions, making it possible to ignore routine self-protective mechanisms, such as hand-washing, avoiding smoke and eating properly.

For those who consider Candidas might be the cause of their sinus condition, alcohol should be eliminated entirely, as it provides a major dietary contributor to Candidas.

STOP SMOKING and avoid secondhand smoke.

The Number One thing anyone can do to treat their sinuses kindly, is to STOP SMOKING. The American Lung Association sponsors free clinics to aid those who want to stop smoking and need assistance to do so. Physicians can provide nicotine patches which will aid the smoker to reduce the craving for nicotine. Help is available if you have tried to quit smoking and just don't seem to be able to do so on your own.

Nicotine paralyzes the cilia, the small hairs within the nose that beat rhythmically to move congestion and mucus out of the respiratory system. Smoke of any kind, and that includes cigar, pipe, campfire and outdoor barbecue fires. Marijuana and cocaine (whether smoked or snorted) are very harmful to the nasal mucous membrane.

At the tissue level, smoke and nicotine cause irritation of the mucous membrane. The worse the condition of the sinuses, the greater the irritation. The more the irritation, the more inflamed the mucous membrane becomes. Inflammation of the mucous membrane results in swelling, increased mucus secretion and further damage to the cilia.

Further, the American Heart Association estimates that secondhand smoke might be a contributing factor in the heart disease deaths of forty thousand nonsmoking Americans every year. Their studies indicate that fifty million nonsmoking adults over the age of thirty-five are exposed to secondhand smoke regularly, and fifty percent of all

American children live in households with one or more smokers, a factor in long-term health risks and additional health care costs.

If the care of your own respiratory system is not enough impetus to stop smoking, secondhand smoke kills approximately four thousand people annually, is particularly harmful to children with asthma and increases the risk of respiratory infections for all those exposed.

Those who are regularly exposed to secondhand smoke should consume foods high in beta-carotene (carrots, squash, yams, sweet potatoes and other yellow-orange vegetables), as well as foods rich in vitamin C (citrus fruits, peppers and broccoli) and vitamin E (wheat germ and nuts) because these antioxidants help the body cleanse the lungs and eliminate pollutants.

Limit caffeine. Although it appears that one or two cups of coffee or cola drinks a day are not harmful, caffeine contributes to feelings of anxiety or jitteriness, and it may possibly stress our immune systems in ways that decrease our stamina. Caffeine raises blood pressure, can create heart rhythm disturbances, stimulates the central nervous system and reduces the depth of sleep (which is known to be harmful to the necessary rest that our immune systems require).

Black or green tea might be an excellent substitute for coffee as a morning beverage. Researchers
have recently found that both black and green tea
raise antioxidant activity in the blood by forty to
fifty percent.

Stop That Cold in its First Stages

Listen to your own self-healing instincts. Illness is
the way your body tells you to slow down. Your
body needs a rest—give it one. Pamper yourself.

Many viruses are responsible for the common
cold. Most colds—up to fifty percent of them—are
caused by one of the more than one hundred se-
rotypes of the rhinoviruses. Pinpointing the specific cause of each one by virus isolation is
impractical. So, rather than attempting to identify
the causative agent among all these viruses, we
should look at what they have in common and
take actions that will help us avoid being infected
by any of them.

Chilling of the body surface does not by itself
induce colds, but it is accepted by the medical
establishment that excessive fatigue, emotional
distress or allergies may facilitate an infection.

Thus, colds and upper respiratory infections
are often the result of life-style habits that de-
press the immune system, making it possible for
that virus to get a foothold in your body.

Smoking, environmental pollutants, a poor diet, rushing around, meeting deadlines, staying out late, eating on the run at some fast food place, not getting proper rest. Does this all sound familiar? Of course it does. All of us do most of these things at some time or another. The reasons sound familiar too, "I just had to get it done," or "If I don't take care of it, no one else will." How about, "But they are all relying on me, I have to get to that meeting," or " I don't have time to cook tonight, I'll grab a sandwich."

If you are serious about taking care of your sinuses, one of your priorities must be prevention: preventing that upper respiratory tract infection before it has your sinuses yelling for help. Just like many other health conditions, it is easier to prevent a cold than to treat it when it has become debilitating.

Rest to Repair

When you feel the first nasal or throat discomfort, be aware. You are beginning to get a cold.

LISTEN TO YOUR BODY!

Don't push yourself. Give yourself time. You need time for your immune system to gear up and respond to the threat. Go to bed early. Immune system functions are elevated when your autonomic nervous system assumes control, and immune-enhancing compounds are released into your system during deep sleep. Virally damaged cells are regenerated between midnight and 4 AM.

If you feel tired, you probably are tired. Let your body rest, slow down, take it easy. If you don't feel up to doing all the things you usually do, everyone will probably survive until you feel better.

Sleep

Sleeplessness can increase anxiety symptoms and interfere with the healing process. Difficulty in sleeping is quite often due to poor bedtime habits or thinking patterns which interfere with the ability to get to sleep. If your sleep is poor or interrupted, or if you waken early feeling fatigued, don't resort to sleeping medications. These medications are habit forming, are only for short-term sleeplessness, and should only be taken after attempts have been made to improve your bedtime habits. Prescription sleeping medications can alter normal sleeping patterns and suppress REM sleep. Try to maintain a healthy internal biological clock by going to bed and arising at the same time each day. Naps are good if they are taken early in the day, for not more than thirty minutes.

Avoid stimulants such as caffeine for three to five hours before bedtime. Avoid alcohol. While you might think of alcohol as a "night cap" or a relaxing drug, even moderate amounts of alcohol can disrupt sleep and often cause a backlash of sleeplessness in the early morning hours.

Herbal sleep formulas in teas, tinctures and capsules are available in most health food stores. Valerian, chamomile, oats, passionflower and balm are the best, according to Varro Tyler, Ph.D., professor of pharmacognosy at Purdue University.

You might want to try melatonin, a normal brain chemical. This is a natural hormonelike compound produced by the pineal gland which resides deep in the brain and other tissues in the body. It is involved in numerous aspects of biological and physiological regulation. It sets and maintains the inner clocks governing the natural rhythms of body functions. Experimentally, melatonin has been shown to modify immunity, the stress response and some aspects of the aging process. Low doses of oral melatonin from 0.1 to 10 mg. have been shown to be a useful aid in insomnia. Naturally, melatonin in the body is lowered in the morning by light, and darkness increases the levels of this chemical which the body uses to regulate sleep cycles.

However, some side effects have been reported such as nightmares, headaches and depression. Research suggests that these side effects are possibly the result of too high a dosage. 1 mg. several times a week appear to be sufficient for the majority of individuals. There is some very preliminary research that suggests those with autoimmune conditions should not use melatonin.

Valerian, an herb, reduces activity in the central nervous system. Hops, another herb, is a digestive tonic and sedative and may help you relax. Dr. Tyler also recommends purchasing dried hops flowers and placing them in a small bag underneath your pillow for additional aid in sleeping as the odor is very soothing.

During the oncoming phase of a cold, you might want to try some herbal treatments. While herbs work slowly, they don't have the extreme side effects of many prescription medications, which do nothing to "cure" a cold, only to suppress symptoms. In fact, traditional drug store cold remedies can make a cold last longer. Because they suppress symptoms, they can halt the body's natural responses, such as detoxification and balancing.

Take 15 to 20 drops of Echinacea extract, a natural immune activator, twice daily.

Try several cups of an herbal tea that will aid in increasing perspiration, to eliminate toxins more rapidly. Peppermint, rose hips, or ginger are just a few you might enjoy. Cayenne and ginger capsules will encourage your body temperature to rise which will aid in the elimination of toxins.

Drink lots of liquids: juice, water, broth.

Bathe—the skin is the largest organ of elimination, and it will perform more efficiently if you have bathed frequently.

Increase your intake of vitamin C. Ester-C form of the vitamin is less likely to cause diarrhea.

Zinc extract drops, or zinc tablet allowed to dissolve in the mouth, create a pH environment that discourages the replication of the virus.

Eat chicken soup. Your mother was right: this has beneficial effects on the cold symptoms by stimulating the release and movement of mucus.

Avoid refined flour, sugar and dairy foods. All of these foods increase mucus production.

Relax. If you are a regular exerciser, take a few days off. Vigorous exercise adds stress to an already stressed immune system. Perhaps you recall Magic Johnson quit his basketball career when he was diagnosed with HIV. This retirement was on the recommendation of his physicians. He did not retire because he might infect others, but because the extremes of exercise professional athletes subject themselves to was thought to be too stressful for his already weakened immune system. While we are not suggesting a common cold is as severe as this killer virus, the principle of avoiding over-stressing the immune system—which now has additional work to do during a cold or the flu—is the same.

It is not necessary to stay in bed. Take a brief and relaxed walk. Enjoy the scenery and do a little deep breathing.

If your nose is stuffy and you cannot sleep, put a little eucalyptus oil in the vaporizer to help clear your nose.

Foods that put a strain on your digestive system should be minimized. Dairy products, fried foods, peanut butter, white flour all tend to cause congestion.

Vegetable juices, green drinks (such as barley grass, chlorella or spirulina) and herbal teas promote mucus elimination, help alkalize the body and rebuild healthy blood. Remember, viruses prefer an acid environment.

Avoid sugars. They create an acid environment (which viruses love) and reduce the ability of white blood cells to do their job.

Eat light nutritious meals.

Avoid the immune suppressors alcohol and nicotine.

Avoid the zinc absorption blocker caffeine.

Extra stress vitamins—the water-soluble vitamins B complex and C with bioflavanoids—are excellent and will help stimulate numerous immune functions.

Vitamin A and carotenes keep the mucous membranes strong and resistant.

Add the antioxidants: Vitamin E, zinc and selenium.

When the acute phase of the cold has passed, add some yogurt with active cultures to repair your intestinal bacteria.

If the cough and sore throat hang on, add six to eight garlic capsules daily. Garlic is an excellent antioxidant and natural antibiotic.

Herbal expectorants are effective, without all the side effects of prescription medications as long as dosages are not exceeded. They can be purchased at a health food store and might contain mullen, ma huang, calendula and ginger.

For the discomfort of aches and pains which sometimes accompany a cold, try white willow bark.

Throat-coating herbal teas are well tolerated by children. Try wild cherry, orange peel, cardamom or ginger.

When you begin to feel better, take an herbal immune activator such as echinacea or astragalus extract. Add zinc-providing herbs to help strengthen your immune system.

Antioxidants—the Green Pastures of Life

How many times our parents encouraged us to eat our vegetables. But why? Because they are good for you. For openers, they are rich in vitamins and minerals, they provide dietary fiber and are low in fat and sodium. In addition, fruits and vegetables are good sources of vitamin C and beta carotene, two well known antioxidants.

Antioxidants need to be part of your life every day. They are substances which unite with oxygen, protecting all the cells of the body and other constituents such as enzymes from being destroyed or modified by oxidation. Oxidants of free radicals can be generated from exposure to environmental factors such as pollution, cigarette smoke, radiation and pesticides.

Dr. Denham Harman, of University of Nebraska College of Medicine, first proposed the theory of free radicals thirty years ago. He believes the proliferation of free radicals within the human body contributes to disease and premature aging, and that good nutrition, moderate daily exercise and the limitation of stress are keys to good health. Dr. Harman proposed free radicals are highly unstable and potentially disruptive molecules the body produces in response to normal cellular metabolism and environmental toxins. Time has shown Dr. Harman's theories to be accurate.

Dr. Jeffrey Blumberg, professor of nutrition and chief of the Antioxidants Research Laboratory of the U.S. Department of Agriculture Human Nutrition Research Center at Tufts University, recently told *The Medical Tribune* there is strong evidence suggesting a role for antioxidant supplementation which comes from the realms of experimental biology. He states antioxidants have been demonstrated in human studies to modulate free-radical damage to DNA and enhance immune responsiveness.

Dr. Victor Herbert, professor of medicine at Mount Sinai School of Medicine in New York, pointed out while the evidence that antioxidants may play an important role in promoting health and reducing the risk of some chronic disease has been accumulating for over thirty years, supplements are not substitutes for a healthy diet.

"One cannot engage in adverse life-styles with smoking, drinking, avoiding exercise, etc., and expect antioxidant supplements to guarantee health," said Dr. Herbert. He added, however, "It is worth appreciating that relative to drug and other medical therapies, nutritional interventions such as antioxidant supplementation is very inexpensive and absolutely safe in recommended doses."

Humans are complex chemical factories, taking in the necessary nutrients to grow and repair every part of the structure, from bone and internal organs to muscle and skin. Oxygen and nutrients are needed to fuel this system daily, and they are taken in from the air we breathe, the liquids we drink and the foods we eat.

Free radicals are the toxic by-products of the use of oxygen in human beings: oxygen that is absolutely essential for life. Free radicals are highly unstable reactive compounds in the body, created by normal metabolism of dietary fats, strenuous exercise and exposure to environmental pollution or radiation. Free radicals, stray atoms with an unpaired electron, roam the body trying to find other compounds to react with and complete themselves. These reactions can destabilize other molecules within the body, leading to the formation of still more free radicals. This process does its damage at the cellular level, altering the way cells encode genetic information and destroying the cells' protective membranes, particularly those of the immune system. The immune system membrane is crucial to the immune response. The membranes, or outer cell walls, have a high content of polyunsaturated fatty acids, and these fats are particularly susceptible to oxidation or free radical damage. Antioxidant enzymes help protect these cell membranes, and are necessary for good immune system health.

Successful prevention of chronic infections depends on controlling this free radical destruction of the cell membrane.

When skin wrinkles, rubber becomes hard and metal rusts, we are seeing examples of oxidation. Oxidation is a toxic by-product of oxygen metabolism. Since we cannot exist without oxygen, oxidation by these free radicals is inevitable. While we cannot stop it entirely, we can do something to limit the amount of damage this process causes to our cells, and protect the immune system. The answer lies in a way to prevent these oxidizing free radical molecules from joining with our cells. We need to provide them with molecules to link up with instead of the cells of the body. These molecules are known as antioxidants, and by connecting with these free radicals they, in effect, neutralize them—preventing them from damaging our cells.

Provide your body with a good variety of antioxidants. Vitamins A, E, and C and selenium are some of the main antioxidant nutrients that can readily be found in any health food store and by eating a varied diet.

A variety of herbs and vitamin supplements are excellent sources, in addition to the sources in a varied diet of fresh fruits and green vegetables.

Herbs—Concentrated Food

Herbs are concentrated foods, edible plants that are safe to take as foods, and are rich in nutrients that can stimulate the body's own healing mechanisms. They can be nourishing, as well as providing minerals that are sometimes lost in foods that are grown in poor soil.

Antioxidant rich herbal extracts include echinacea, Siberian ginseng, pau d'arco, red clover, ginkgo biloba and spirulina.

Sea vegetable nutrients and herbal sources of bioflavonoids are support factors you can use and enjoy to maintain optimum immune response. Herbal drinks are unique, all-natural means of providing the optimum absorbable nutrients, in addition to aiding in maintaining the proper acid-alkaline balance of the blood.

Japanese green tea has received a lot of positive publicity in the U.S. for its polyphenol activity reported to prevent skin cancers and tumor growth, and to aid in the reduction of heart disease through the reduction of serum cholesterol levels. In the Orient, this green tea has been used for centuries as a bronchodilator, and it now has been found to have antioxidant and anti-allergen flavonoids.

Una da gato, or cat's claw, is another antioxidant from the Peruvian rain forest that has shown excellent results in enhancing immunity and increasing resistance to respiratory ailments.

Many drugs use plant isolates and concentrates, but herbs are not drugs. Herbs are whole nutrients that support the body in its work of healing and restoration of health.

Drugs often treat only the symptoms, and sometimes provide immediate relief that seems miraculous. With herbs, you need to be patient. They work through the glands and the cells, at the deepest levels of body chemistry. For that reason, it may seem that they take longer or that they are not doing anything. Be patient, give herbs time. Most people feel some improvement with herbal treatments in about six days.

Sometimes herbs get some bad press. That bad press is often not because of the herbs, but because of the use people make of them. For example, ingredient panels on some recently notorious "herbal high" products list ma huang, Chinese ephedra, Ephedra sinica, ephedra extract, epitonin or ephedrine. These ephedrine-containing products bear labels that appear to be targeted at adolescents and young adults and imply that the product can produce feelings of euphoria, sexual awareness, or even cosmic consciousness! The labels often portray the products as apparent alternatives to illegal street drugs such as "ecstacy." Sold in night clubs, novelty and "head shops," as well as the Internet, these products sometimes contain many, many times the recommended dosages of herbs.

As with anything else, common sense and safety should be foremost in the use of any product, whether it is bought in a health food store, a pharmacy, or recommended by a physician.

Dosages of herbal treatments for children should always be reduced. A baby will only need 1/8th of the amount given an adult and up to half of the adult dose is appropriate for a teenager.

Phytochemicals—Immune System Enhancers

Fruits and vegetables provide more than antioxidants, they provide phytochemicals, compounds existing naturally in all plant foods *(phyto* is the Greek word for plant). They are not vitamins or minerals. They have no known nutritional value, yet they are associated with prevention and treatment of at least four of the leading causes of death—cancer, heart disease, diabetes and hypertension.

Phytochemicals give plant foods their color, odor and flavor, and there are thousands of them in a single food. The average tomato contains up to 10,000 phytochemicals alone. Over the past several years, scientists have discovered more than fourteen classes of phytochemicals in the foods we eat, and the numbers are still growing.

Phytochemicals go by names like indoles, isothiocyanates, isoflavones, and genistein, and they boast a variety of health benefits. Some have been shown to enhance the immune system while others lower serum cholesterol.

Certain phytochemicals, the isothiocyanates, for example, have the ability to trigger formation of enzymes that can protect cells of the body against damage from a variety of damaging oxidants. At present, numerous studies are being conducted using phytochemicals individually, in various combinations, or in combination with other nutrients to discover their role in disease prevention.

The National Cancer Institute and American

Heart Association recommend a diet that includes at least five servings daily of fruits and vegetables. It doesn't matter whether fruits and vegetables are fresh, frozen or canned. The fresher the vegetables, the more nutrients; since freezing preserves phytochemicals, frozen vegetables may be better than raw ones that sit in the refrigerator too long, according to Dr. Julie Albrecht, Associate Director of Nutritional Sciences at the University of Nebraska.

Supplements containing phytochemicals are now becoming very popular, and scientific advances have isolated and concentrated the most active phytonutrients, but at the present, scientists feel that the large variety of combined phytonutrients available in the whole fruit or vegetable is far more beneficial than supplementation.

Dr. Herbert says, "Just taking vitamin C is not synonymous with fruits and vegetables. People who eat large amounts of fruits and vegetables have high blood levels of a host of phytochemicals and antioxidants, one of which is vitamin C."

Diet—For Overall Health

Hippocrates, the great Greek physician, is not only the father of medicine but the father of practical nutrition. One of his most famous statements is, "Let thy food by thy medicine."

Everyone knows the expression: "You are what you eat." The very tissues of your body, the fuels that power every cell, the hormones that keep all your glandular functions operating, all must ultimately be furnished by the foods you eat.

In the 1700s, Dr. James Lind discovered the terrible disease that made so many sailors ill on long voyages, scurvy, could be prevented by addition of citrus fruit to their diets, although the necessary ingredient—ascorbic acid or vitamin C—was not identified for another 200 years.

As we become more aware of the effects of diet on our overall health, with reports from the American Medical Association, the Centers for Disease Control, the American Heart Association and others on how diet affects cholesterol, blood pressure, heart disease, arthritis and dozens of other chronic conditions, it is easy to see sinus health can easily be made worse or better by diet.

There are specific factors in any diet aimed at improving the condition of the sinuses, such as things that contribute to mucus formation.

It is well documented that milk and dairy products contribute to the increase and thickening of mucus secretions and should be minimized or eliminated. Calcium, an important part of any diet, can be replaced from sources other than dairy. Broccoli, kale, sesame seeds, sesame seed butter, tofu, sea vegetables and soy cheese all have high concentrations of calcium.

Oriental diets contain almost no dairy products, but are high in soy products. Those populations do not suffer from a number of diseases linked to calcium deficiencies, such as osteoporosis, in the numbers that plague the U.S. population.

Calcium/magnesium supplementation in combination can be purchased in any health food store. An adequate daily dose for the adult female is 1,200 mg. calcium and 500 mg. of magnesium. Calcium and magnesium should be taken in combination as the magnesium is essential for the metabolism of the calcium.

To achieve a balanced, nutritionally sound diet you need to select foods that are:

low in fat,

low in sugar and,

high in fiber.

If you follow these three concepts, you will not need to worry about cholesterol, saturated fats or calories. A balanced diet is important because it underlies every other nutritional consideration. A diet which contains a variety of foods is absolutely necessary in order to get the full variety of nutrients. No single food or group of foods contains everything we need in order to be healthy.

Experts at the U.S. Department of Agriculture have constructed what they describe as a daily food guide pyramid (Fig. 5), with six food groups, rather than the previous division of four food groups. They have indicated that you need to start at the wide base of the pyramid with plenty from the group of breads, cereals, rice and pasta (6-11 servings); the vegetable group (3-5 servings) and fruit group (2-4 servings). This pyramid includes the milk, yogurt and cheese group (2-3 servings) which, for someone with sinusitis, should be replaced with soy products, as in the Traditional healthy Asian diet pyramid (Fig. 6).

Figure 5

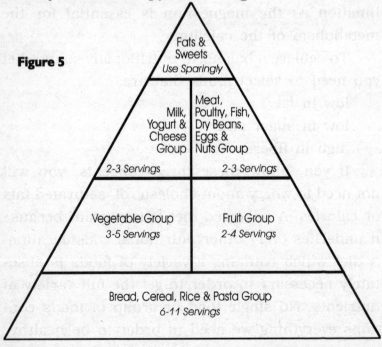

Fats &
Sweets
Use Sparingly

Milk,
Yogurt &
Cheese
Group
2-3 Servings

Meat,
Poultry, Fish,
Dry Beans,
Eggs &
Nuts Group
2-3 Servings

Vegetable Group
3-5 Servings

Fruit Group
2-4 Servings

Bread, Cereal, Rice & Pasta Group
6-11 Servings

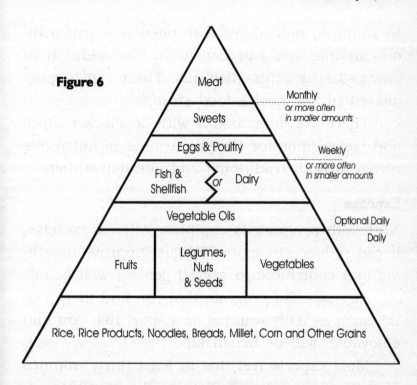

Figure 6

In this alternative pyramid, rice, corn, noodles, millet, breads and other grains form the base of the diet, followed by fruits, legumes, nuts, seeds and vegetables. Dairy foods are not part of the healthy, traditional diets of Asia, and many nutritional experts feel that this diet is far more beneficial than the typical diet of the average American.

Chinese people get eleven percent of their protein from animal products and eighty-nine percent from plants; Americans, on the other hand, derive seventy percent of their protein from animal products and thirty percent from plants.

In addition, individuals with postnasal drip without an infection can benefit by the addition of omega-3 fatty acids—fish oils. These can be purchased in any health food store.

There are many books with delicious recipes and suggestions for the preparation of nutritious meals in both traditional and alternative diets.

Exercise

No health program is complete without exercise. It can reduce stress and fatigue, improve breathing and contribute to overall general well being.

Any exercise program that you find therapeutic, such as daily walking or a sport that you find enjoyable, will be beneficial.

Most experts feel that at least thirty minutes four times a week can improve the physical condition and health of anyone.

Consider Allergy

If you eliminate smoking, along with alcohol and caffeine, follow the above diet for a period of month, and still and do not find that your sinus condition is improved, then it might be time to consider allergies. For the next several weeks, eliminate those foods that have been shown to most frequently produce allergic reactions which might be part of the cause of your sinusitis.

The frequent offenders:

Wheat and grain products

Chocolate

White sugar

Corn products

Brewer's and baker's yeast

Citrus fruits

Foods in the nightshade groups
  (such as potatoes and eggplant)

Tomatoes

Bell peppers

Eggs

Shellfish

Nuts

Peanuts

Food colorings
  (read the labels of the products you
  normally use)

If your condition has not improved after removing
these items from your diet for several weeks, it
may be time to try an elimination diet.

The quick steps—How to perform an elimination diet

List the foods you suspect are causing
your symptoms.

Abstain from five foods on this list for
a full five days.

At the end of these five days, reintroduce the suspected foods one at a time and note your reaction as follows:

> Take your resting pulse and then eat a substantial, unseasoned portion of the suspect food, by itself, as the first food of the day.

> Fifteen minutes later, take your pulse again and every fifteen minutes for the next hour and a half.

> The majority of symptoms will appear within six hours after eating.

> Test the foods on your list using this method—one each day.

If you find foods are causing allergic reactions and contributing to the condition of your sinuses, eliminate them and substitute others that contribute the same elements to your diet.

Water—the Essential Nutrient

Water is essential to all bodily functions. It is necessary for our kidneys to remove waste products, and it is vital for digestion and the metabolism of all the nutrients we eat. It carries nutrients and oxygen to the cells in the body through the blood. It aids in regulation of body temperature, it lubricates our joints, and it is essential for healthy sinuses as it lubricates the mucous membranes of the respiratory system.

The human body is approximately eighty percent water. Without a daily intake of water, we find ourselves with reduced blood volume. The result of that is there are less oxygen and fewer nutrients being transported to all the cells of the body. Lack of water results in constipation, muscle soreness and water retention because the body retains the water already in the cells in order to compensate for the lack of water intake.

A healthy adult should drink about eight to ten 8-ounce glasses of water daily, spread throughout the day. Coffee, tea, soft drinks and fruit juice are not substitutes for water. Although all these things contain water, they also contain other ingredients that can possibly block some of water's benefits.

Herbal teas and soups are two of the ways you can increase your intake of water if you find it difficult to drink this much plain water. However, many people find that, with a concentrated effort to take in more water, after a week or so they are able to drink the eight to ten glasses without difficulty.

Add moisture to the air you breathe, whether by adding a humidifier to your air conditioner/

furnace or by a vaporizer in your bedroom. Pay attention to the moisture content of the air you breathe.

If air travel is a frequent necessity, be sure to increase your water intake during the flight as the air on planes is notoriously dry. You might also want to take along a spritz bottle and spray your face several times. It will not only benefit your sinuses, it will keep moisture in your skin as well.

Sinus irrigation, by instilling warm, salinated water into one nostril at a time, is one of the least harmful ways, with the exception of internal lubrication by drinking water, to add moisture to the mucous membranes.

Rest—the Ease Restorer

Lack of sleep has been documented to lower immunity. It helps to be physically comfortable, mentally at ease. Sleep will be better in a freshly made bed in a well ventilated and dust-free environment. If you sleep poorly, or your sleep is interrupted or you waken feeling fatigued, you are limiting the ability of your immune system to repair itself since most of the repair of the immune system takes place during sleep.

Avoid stimulants (such as caffeine) for three to five hours before bedtime. Avoid alcohol. While many think of alcohol as a relaxing drug, even moderate amounts can disrupt sleep and often cause a backlash of sleeplessness in the early morning hours.

Try an herbal tea such as chamomile, valerian, passion flower, rosemary, scullcap as a natural sedative.

Make the bedroom inviting to sleep in. Make the window treatments heavy enough to keep light and noise out.

Establish a bedtime routine by setting up a conditioned response. If you regularly wash your face, brush your teeth, set out your clothing for the next day, wind the clock, walk the dog; do all these things in a regular, routine order. This will become your conditioned response that triggers your body to go to sleep after these things are completed. Whatever activities you choose for your conditioned response, such as a hot bath, praying or meditating, remember to choose only relaxing activities. Avoid anxiety-arousing activities such as paying bills, watching horror movies or listening to loud, energizing music.

If you go to bed and find that you cannot fall asleep, do not stay in bed worrying. After no more than twenty minutes, get up, do something that you regularly find relaxing in some other part of the house. Read or watch television, or do some other quiet activity, until you begin to feel sleepy. Only then should you go back to bed.

Exercise just before attempting to sleep will interfere with sleep. Three to five hours before bedtime, heavy exercise will interfere with your ability to sleep. However, light exercise, such as a walk around the block after dinner, will improve the amount of good refreshing sleep you will get in the early part of the night.

If you have been unable to sleep and then find that you are very sleepy in the middle of the afternoon of the next day, change your activity. Get out of your chair, move, stretch. Drink a cup of refreshing herbal tea or take a water break rather than a cigarette break.

Researchers have identified two types of sleep: light and heavy. During the lighter sleep, known as REM or rapid eye movement, you release stress and tension as you dream. During the heavier sleep, called non-REM, your body's healing mechanisms go into action, repairing cellular damage, rebuilding structures torn down during exercise, repairing your immune system.

Avoid relying on sleeping medications, which are not only habit forming, but have many disagreeable side effects. Instead, practice some meditation techniques, take a warm relaxing bath or perform deep breathing.

According to Dr. Deepak Chopra—a practicing endocrinologist and founding president of the American Association of Ayurvedic Medicine, the bestselling author of a number of health books, who has introduced America to this ancient Eastern system of Medicine—the ideal bedtime for the deepest sleep and for being in sync with your natural biorhythms, is before 9 PM. According to this system of medicine, the eight hours of sleep that begin at 9:30 PM are twice as beneficial and restful as the hours of sleep in the early morning.

Stress—the Killer "Virus"

Worry and anxiety can be as detrimental to your health as any virus. That stress can be anything that triggers your fight-or-flight response. However, the effects of stress can be both positive and negative. Positive stress is the excitement an experienced performer feels just before a performance. In this case, the adrenaline response improves the performance.

Negative stress can be short-term (such as the fear, pressure, and need for quick decisions when the driver in the car in front of you suddenly slams on the brakes), or long-term (such as the stress you might feel in a complex, high pressure job). Too much stress, especially over a long period of time, can drain energy, cause undue wear and tear on the body, and make an individual vulnerable to illness, premature aging and psychological breakdown.

Photographs of presidents when they entered office and when they left, sometimes only a matter of four years, provide a vivid example of the toll a high-stress occupation can take on the body and appearance.

We can divide stress into two major types: physical stress and psychological stress. Physical stress is created by demands on the body such as those caused by accidents, illness, lack of sleep, chemical toxins, a demanding work schedule, or prolonged psychological stress. Psychological stress is created by mental or emotional demands on the body. Psychological stress can be simply the result of physical stress. However, psychological stress is more often caused by mental or emotional demands from your personal beliefs, family, work or friends. Such stresses can be time pressures, frustration of blocked desires, the conflict of having to make choices, and anxiety, which is the response to a perceived threat.

It is well documented that stress can affect the immune system. Stressful situations are all around each of us, each and every day. We can choose how we respond to the daily stresses. Once the stress overwhelms us, we become fatigued and can then develop stress-related conditions, such as sinusitis.

The flight-or-flight response, that dramatic reaction that prepares us to fight or run when threatened, causes physiological changes which include an elevation in blood pressure, heart rate, respiration, metabolism, epinephrine production, blood glucose, peripheral vascular constriction and pupil dilation, to name a few. Continual, unrelieved stress, with these constant physiological changes produced by the flight-or-flight response, sometimes results in physical symptoms as the weakest part of our body becomes vulnerable and finally breaks down.

Stress Management

Hundreds of studies show a strong correlation between the chemical changes, physical changes and emotional responses to stress and a patient's symptoms. While you might find it difficult to think of stress as being related to your sinusitis, you can probably recall the last time you got a cold after you stayed out late at night, missed meals, hurried around trying to do too many errands in one afternoon. Take that idea one step further and recognize that the cold often was soon followed by a sinus infection.

Almost forty years ago Drs. T. Holmes and R. Rahe developed the Social Readjustment Scale which demonstrated that individuals who had significant social change within the last year—such as loss of a loved one, change of job, marriage, retirement, pregnancy, business readjustment—had an eighty percent chance of developing an illness.

Be aware of your stressors. When you identify the situations that precipitate tension for you, identify the muscles you tighten in response and take steps to consciously relax them.

Breathing is a powerful way to energize and relax. Try some simple deep breathing, particularly when you are angry or tired.

Yoga is an ancient method of relaxation, breathing, meditation and mind/body control which you might find beneficial in keeping stress at bay.

If you find yourself repeating doom-and-gloom statements to yourself on a regular basis, it is no wonder that you are stressed out. Defeatist, negative thinking makes us feel terrible, and it robs us of vitality and creativity. It may sound Pollyannaish to make positive statements to yourself such as, "I'm am healthy," or "My life gets better every day," but those who practice it say it is quite beneficial in improving their mood and keeping stress away.

Relaxation skills are just like any other: they improve with practice. By the active tightening and releasing of gross muscle groups, noting the differences between sensations of tension and relaxation, you will soon increase your ability to identify tension and actively reduce it. Try relaxation/self-hypnosis tapes or biofeedback as part of a stress reduction program.

If you are following a nutritious diet, be sure it includes sufficient amounts of the B vitamins, and calcium, the nutrients that repair the nerves.

Avoidance of Triggers

Avoidance of triggering substances in any sinus health program is the single most effective, least expensive and least complicated option to consider. Pollens, dust, dust mites, mold spores, dogs, cats, smoke, chemical agents, aerosols, or anything else you are aware of that aggravates your condition should be eliminated or controlled as much as possible. Most of us would rather take a pill, get an injection, find a doctor who will finally DO something to help us rather than take an avoidance step—even though it has been found that avoidance of triggering substances works well and can be one of the first steps toward wellness.

Dust

Household dust is the accumulated debris of your environment. It is a mixture of dust, pollen, various fibers, insect parts, pesticides, hair and shed skin cells—and it is everywhere in your home. These factors need to be considered and controlled. Usually it is not just one thing, such as pollen or dust mites. Although it is not possible to live in a sterile and dust-free environment, you can do a lot to limit your exposure.

Focus your preliminary efforts on the bedroom, where you spend approximately one-third of your time.

Clear the room. Remove everything: furniture, drapes, curtains, clothing and carpeting.

Have the room thoroughly cleaned and then clean the furniture that has been removed. Asthmatics and those who are quite aware that house dust is a factor in their condition, should return to the room only that furniture which is essential.

Pillowcases, mattresses and bed coverings that are allergy-free are available from such sources as

Allergy Free Inc. (1-800-ALLERGY), the Self Care Catalog (1-800-345-3771) or a local medical supply house in your area.

Ceiling fans not only harbor dust on their wide blades, they add it to the mix of allergens in a room by recirculating dust-laden air. Fans should be cleaned regularly, particularly if they are directly over the bed.

Store only frequently used clothing in the closet. Place this clothing in airtight, zipper-sealed vinyl clothing storage bags.

If you must do your own cleaning, inexpensive dust masks can be purchased in any drugstore.

Wash bedding frequently.

Establish a routine for regular cleaning of the bedroom.

Install an air filter which can effectively clear the air of pollen, dust, mold spores and animal allergens. Be sure that you purchase one that is adequate to filter the air in the entire room. These are available from a variety of sources, such as Sears, the catalogues mentioned or air conditioning suppliers.

Dust Mites

Dust mites just love carpeting. It is their most favorite place to make their home. Carpet removal from the bedroom will limit your exposure to them and the symptoms they cause. For those who find removing the carpeting is not an option, Acarosan powder can be of benefit. This product kills the mites for removal by vacuuming. It is available from your pharmacist without a prescription.

Cockroaches

For reasons which are yet unclear, black children are three times more allergic to cockroaches and their residue than whites. Inner city living may be part of the cause, but even if the conditions of the household in which these children live are kept scrupulously clean, asthma can be triggered by this household pest.

If this pest is pinpointed as the trigger in your asthma, allergy or sinusitis, it is suggested that you inspect the kitchens where you or your child frequently eat, at home or the school cafeteria, and take steps to ensure that all health department regulations concerning cleanliness are met.

Cats and Dogs

Obviously the easiest way to avoid the allergens from pets is to not have one. That may be impossible, for obvious reasons. If the family would rather get rid of you than the beloved family pet, the next best thing is to provide ways to diminish the allergens.

A weekly bath in distilled water can reduce the allergen in cat saliva. Dogs should be bathed regularly also, and their bedding washed and aired frequently. Pets who go outdoors frequently often bring in pollen and other outside potential allergens, and it might be helpful to confine the animals to the house or to certain rooms in the house.

Children can often be satisfied with fish or small reptiles as pets. It is well known that these creatures are seldom allergy-producing.

A special central air and heating system with filters can be helpful in removing these allergens from the air.

Mold

Mold spores prefer to live in dark and dampness. They can grow readily on fruits and vegetables in your refrigerator, on bread, old books, storage boxes, showers, clothes hampers, humidifiers, central air conditioning systems, and even the containers of indoor plants. Look around your living environment, see those places which might be friendly to the growth of mold, dry them out and light them up—you'll feel better very soon if mold is creating your problems.

Avoid places where humidity is likely to be high, such as basements, greenhouses, stables or caves.

Carpeting, including padding, which has been wetted, should be replaced.

Lights in the basement or in closets which are kept on at all times will aid in decreasing mold growth.

Check your ventilation system. You may need to have your duct system professionally cleaned, particularly if your home is over ten years old.

Garbage cans need to be washed out with hot water and bleach frequently.

Outside your house, keep the trees trimmed so that areas of the yard are not very shady most of the time.

Don't allow leaves to accumulate or water to stand in low spots around your house.

Dog kennels, compost piles: these are the types of places where mold spores can flourish and be brought into the house by the residents. They need to be dried out often to prevent mold spore growth.

Pollen

Pollen is everywhere, so unless you are planning to move to the North Pole or Mount Everest, you can hardly avoid it.

Know what pollens affect you and, if possible, stay indoors during that pollen season.

When you are driving, use the air recirculation system in your car and keep the windows closed.

If your problem is grass or trees, have someone else do the yard work during the worst of the season. Limit your outdoor activities during this time.

Place a filter on your air conditioning system, one that filters out small particles, and clean or change it frequently. It is only as good as its ability to perform, and it cannot do the work if it is already clogged with particles. During high allergy seasons, tend to the filter weekly.

Talk to your allergist. Be aware of the pollen count in places you plan to visit before traveling.

A Healthy Indoor Environment

A healthy indoor environment takes action against the indoor pollutants—pollen, mold, plant spores, dust mites, bacteria and viruses. Those most harmful to the respiratory tract are less than one micron in size and are free-floating in the air.

Although it is not always possible to do much about the outdoor air, or that of the office or the work place, most people spend a large portion of their time at home or in the bedroom of that home. For anyone with sinus or other breathing difficulties, it is essential steps be taken to make that air as pollution-free as possible. There are a number of books available on the subject which might give additional information on making the air in your home as healthy as possible. *The Nontoxic Home and Office* by Debra L. Dadd and *The Healthy House* by John Bower are just a couple you might want to read if you are serious about improving the air quality in indoor environments.

Air cleaning and improved ventilation are the best steps you can take to improve the air quality in your home. Air cleaning devices can include furnace filters and portable units. The efficiency of an air cleaner is indicated by the ability to filter a certain percentage of a certain size of free-floating particle. The HEPA filter (high efficiency particulate arrestor) should remove ninety-seven percent of all the 0.3 micron or larger particulates, and can be purchased at many hardware stores or through specialty stores and dealerships dealing in air filters and air conditioning units.

Ventilation duct cleaning is an essential part of any environmental treatment of your home. If you have a high efficiency filter on your furnace or your air conditioning unit, that air still must travel through the ducts of your house.

If you have a free standing unit, it still must handle the air that travels through the duct system and must work harder to keep even a small area clean of particulates.

Companies who perform this service can be located in the Yellow Pages under "Air Conditioning or Furnaces."

Negative Ions

Negative ion generators were designed to restore a natural level of negative ions to indoor areas. These generators work by positively charging smaller particles (dust, smoke, pollen) and then alternatively charged plates attract and retain the charged dirt particles down to 0.01 microns.

Negative ion generators which produce too many negative ions can cause a significant quantity of pollutants to fall onto other grounded surfaces, such as walls or drapes, resulting in a buildup of dirty residue. If you purchase a negative ion generator, it should indicate it cleans the air up to 0.01 microns of particulates and maintains an ideal level of negative ions.

Sears, as well as air conditioner dealerships and Allergy-Free and Self-Care, provides negative ion generators on their electronic air cleaning and filtering systems.

Household Plants

Plants are efficient oxygenators, filters and humidifiers. They remove the carbon dioxide we exhale, add moisture to the air and improve the quality of indoor air. The Foliage for Clean Air Council recommends a minimum of two plants per one hundred square feet of floor space in a home with eight to ten foot ceilings.

The most common organic chemical in the average indoor environment is formaldehyde. It is released from a variety of plastics and synthetic carpeting, upholstery and foam padding.

According to the EPA, chrysanthemums, dwarf date palms and Boston ferns are excellent for removing formaldehyde from the air.

Spider plants are useful to remove carbon monoxide.

Areca palms filter xylene.

English ivy filters benzene.

Aloe vera, philodendron and ficus reduce the levels of a variety of pollutants produced by household chemicals.

Radon

Radon is the product of the natural decay of uranium found in rocks and in the earth's crust. It seeps into buildings through holes and cracks. The Centers for Disease Control and Prevention, and the American Lung Association, contend that radon causes thousands of preventable lung cancer deaths each year. When combined with smoking, radon can be an especially serious health risk. Although none of these studies looked at the effects of this gas on the sinuses, something this hazardous to the lungs cannot be beneficial to any other body structure.

Salt Lake City-based engineering consultant Vern Rogers and his colleagues analyzed radon's diffusion through samples of residential concrete. They found molecules of radon gas passed through two to four inch thick samples of concrete. Since radon is an odorless and colorless gas, and most air cleaners do not remove it from the air, it is suggested you have your home tested for it. Kits are available for do-it-yourself testing, and if radon is found, basement cracks should be sealed and basement ventilation improved.

Candida Albicans—Something to Consider

If you find that changing your diet, stopping smoking and all the other things suggested do not end your suffering, you might consider that it is no longer a virus or bacteria but a yeast infection. As mentioned previously, this is a controversial issue, but you might want to consider it before you decide it is not your problem.

Dr. William Crook, a prolific medical writer and lecturer, has said: "The road to better health will not be found through more drugs, doctors, and hospitals. Instead it will be found through better nutrition and changes in life-style."

Dr. Crook, author of *The Yeast Connection*, feels this common yeast may be responsible for many cases of sinusitis because it causes a dysfunction of the immune system. He states *Candida albicans* can wear down the immune system, making it possible for viral infections to take hold.

Yeast is a fungus that is found on food, in the air and on the exposed surfaces of almost everything. This one is a single-cell fungus, and normally lives in our intestines and mouth, and in the vagina of females. Ordinarily it is kept under control by the good bacteria that live within our bodies. These good or friendly bacteria help in normal bowel function and digestion. As long as the yeast and the friendly bacteria stay in balance we are well. When they get out of balance, then we have a problem.

According to Dr. Crook, the overuse of antibiotics has created a condition whereby the good bacteria are killed along with the bad ones, and that is what has caused the problem.

Millions of women have found themselves with an itchy vaginal yeast infection after a course of antibiotics. Hormones, especially progesterone, have been found to stimulate the growth of Candida. Anything that weakens the immune system can contribute to yeast overgrowth. Chemotherapy, stress, a great variety of medications, illness, environmental toxins and pesticides: all provide an environment where Candida thrive.

Once overgrowth of Candida begins, this fungus feeds on sugar, its favorite food. It can then invade the tissues of the gastrointestinal tract, eventually enter the bloodstream and be carried throughout distant parts of the body with the most favorable environment for growth. Candida just loves the moist mucous membranes of the body. The greatest risk from Candida results from the toxins released during its metabolic processes. These toxins are damaging to the immune system by inhibiting the function of lymphocytes, the blood cells responsible for antibody production. In a complicated chemical process, the toxins from the yeast create a condition whose main symptom is exhaustion/fatigue. Other symptoms follow: sleep disorders, persistent headache, cold extremities, aching, chills, irritability, depression and more. The list of symptoms and disorders blamed on Candida is long: including Chronic Fatigue Syndrome, as well as sinusitis.

Dr. Crook believes that yeast infections can be successfully treated with a special diet and antifungal medications. The treatment depends upon the degree of yeast overgrowth and the extent to which that overgrowth has disabled the immune system. Treatment begins with antifungal medication to kill the overgrowth of the Candida; then elimination of the food for the growth through a controlled diet, which consists primarily of protein and fresh vegetables and limits carbohydrates and sugar; next, restoring normal bacterial flora in the gastrointestinal tract; and then strengthening the immune system.

Physicians, homeopathic practitioners, and others who are confirmed believers in the yeast connection point out that it often takes months and sometimes as long as a year for the health of someone suffering with an overgrowth of yeast to feel better. That takes a commitment to a diet and other stringent health practices which are sometimes difficult to follow.

For those interested in knowing more about this controversial condition and its diagnosis and treatment, there are several books that might be informative: *The Yeast Syndrome* by Trowbridge and Morton; *Back to Health: A Comprehensive Medical and Nutritional Yeast Control Program* by Dennis Remington and Barbara Higa; and Dr. Crook's well-known publication, *The Yeast Connection*, which is available at most health food stores as well as many book stores.

Folk Remedies—You Might Want to Try

Folk remedies come from a variety of sources. They come from your grandmother or some one else's grandmother. Folk medicine is made up of tried-and-true but untested methods. It is not unusual for some ancient remedy or a folk medicine to have some merit. New scientific research validates some of the traditional folk remedies such as willow for pain, sugar to heal wounds, gold for arthritis, and garlic for heart conditions.

There are no real experts in folkloric medicine; there are millions of participants and practitioners throughout the world who have found that something which worked for their parents still works for them.

Some remedies have been handed down through the centuries and remain in current wisdom because they had some basis in science, and some because they attained a mystical connection to a belief system. For whatever reason, they are seldom sufficiently valid to be relied on completely, and no one should forgo basic medical care to rely exclusively on folk medicine. Sometimes they are fun and sometimes they are surprising—most of them are harmless.

Honey

During an attack of sinusitis, chew a one-inch square of honeycomb (available in most health food stores). After you swallow the honey, continue chewing the waxy gum for about ten minutes.

Lemon peel

Sweeten a teaspoonful of grated orange or lemon peel and eat this mixture twice daily.

Fenugreek

Prepare fenugreek seed tea by steeping a teaspoon of the seed in a cup of just boiled water. Allow to steep for about seven minutes and drink.

Ginkgo biloba

Purchase the leaves of this tree (in the herb section of most health food stores). Crush a handful, boil and inhale the vapors. It is possible to prepare this inhalant with gingko from capsules, if the leaves are unavailable.

Ice

Apply an ice pack to the bridge of the nose and across the cheeks. Remove after a few minutes, allow the skin of your face to rewarm and then reapply until you feel some relief.

Salt water

Prepare one cup of warm distilled water with 1/4 teaspoon of sea salt. Leaning over the sink, sniff the solution through one nostril at a time. Do not swallow, but allow the solution to drain out through your mouth. Repeat several times daily and gently blow your nose after each session.

Steam

Stand in a hot shower and breathe. Or lean over a pan full of steaming water with a towel draped over your head to form a tent and inhale. Apply a warm washcloth over your eyes and cheekbones. Repeat. Or use a heating pad or hot water bottle placed across your forehead for fifteen to twenty minutes after steaming.

Aromatherapy

Eucalyptus, lavender, lemon, peppermint, mint or thyme, heated slightly and inhaled can be beneficial. Blend together several drops of rosemary, thyme and peppermint, put on a tissue and inhale.

Hot beverages

A cup of hot coffee, tea or soup can be useful. Cup your hands over the top and sniff the steam from the hot beverage. This can be helpful when you are at work and find your nose is stuffy.

Nose blowing

Only blow one side at a time to prevent pressure buildup which can send bacteria further back into your sinuses.

Spicy foods

Garlic makes mucus less sticky; horseradish contains a chemical similar to one found in decongestants, and cayenne pepper contains a substance that may act as a natural decongestant.

Crush 1 clove of garlic into 1/4 cup of water. With an eyedropper place 10 drops into each nostril, 3 times a day for 3 days.

Take 2 garlic pills and 2 parsley pills every 4 hours while awake for 6 days.

Horseradish

Grate horseradish and gently inhale the vapors.

Mix some grated horseradish with lemon juice and eat 1 teaspoonful 1 hour before breakfast and 1 hour after dinner.

Swallow a tiny bit of Oriental horseradish (available in most sushi restaurants).

If your symptoms vary and you wish to use something that refers specifically to that symptom, try the following:

Coughing

Take several teaspoonfuls of wild cherry bark syrup (available at most health food stores).

Gargle with warm salt water. Do *not* swallow.

Drink warm lemon juice and honey.

Fatigue

Light exercise, several hours before bedtime.

Pace your activities so you do not become overly tired.

Evaluate your vitamins and minerals to be sure you are getting sufficient nutrients.

If fatigue persists, have a physical checkup to rule out other causes.

Headache

Drink 8-10 glasses of water daily to thin mucus.

Install an air cleaner and negative ion generator in your sleeping area.

Use a humidifier to provide steam. Add eucalyptus oil or other aromatic herbs to the water.

Runny nose

Drink 8-10 glasses of water daily to thin secretions.

Use a saline spray to reduce secretions.

Increase your intake of vitamin C to 6,000 mg. daily.

Sore throat

Gargle with warm salt water.

Take garlic capsules 2 times daily. Odor-free garlic is available from health food stores.

Gargle with lemon juice and honey. This is a standard treatment used by professional singers to ease the throat.

Stuffy nose

Increase water intake to 8-10 glasses daily.

Drink hot tea with lemon.

Eat hot chicken soup.

Use steam with herbs added, such as eucalyptus.

Avoid dairy products which increase mucus production.

Avoid wheat, rye, oats and barley.

If the stuffy nose is persistent it might be time to see an allergist.

Wheezing

Avoid gluten and all sulfites (read labels on all foods, particularly prepared meats such as sausages or hot dogs).

Avoid dairy products.

Avoid caffeine.

Drink mint tea several times a day and add 25 drops of lobelia extract.

Thymus
A Long Ignored Part of the Immune System

The thymus gland is a mass of lymphatic tissue situated behind the breastbone or sternum. The role of the thymus is to teach cells how to produce antibodies.

Although many believe that once the thymus has done its work of teaching cells it begins to dissolve into fat and connective tissue, new research indicates that the thymus continues to repair and make immune-responsive cells, when needed.

Believing that the thymus can be stimulated to continue to teach new cells the work of aiding the immune system, several practitioners have suggested that a light tapping of the breastbone for several seconds daily can stimulate this gland.

Why not try it? If it does nothing, it is a harmless exercise; it might be a good time to associate with that exercise a reinforcing reminder to perform some other beneficial health practice. So...tap your thymus—and at the same time rededicate yourself to eat your veggies or stop smoking.

A Few Additional Helpful Hints

Sleeping

Try sleeping in a more upright position by elevating your head on several pillows. This allows the sinuses to continue to drain. Avoid lying down during the day.

Dry cleaning

Air out dry-cleaned garments for several hours before wearing them, as the chemicals can be irritating to the sinuses.

Blankets

Use synthetic rather than wool.

Toilet paper

Avoid scented toilet paper and tissues.

Perfume

Carry a handkerchief with you at all times, so you can use it when needed as a temporary air filter to cover your nose when you are unexpectedly assaulted by irritating scents.

Section V

The Search for Perfect Health

We would all choose to have perfect health if we could. Every day we come in contact with millions of viruses, bacteria, allergens and fungi, and more likely than not, we do not get sick. Our bodies, our minds and our immune systems control and overpower those viruses, bacteria, allergens and fungi. Usually, we think nothing at all about this fact; we just assume that we are going to remain well and most of us are annoyed at our bodies when they fail us and we get a cold or a digestive upset. In fact, we should stand back in constant awe at this wonderful body that is able to keep us well most of the time.

You might find in seeking help that, unfortunately, managed care (HMOs, PPOs)—as structured by medical insurance companies—is built on cost-effective medicine. Many of these organizations insist that all patients must first been seen by a primary care physician and, if they want a further referral, that physician must make such a referral. These physicians are overwhelmed by too many patients and, unfortunately, at the present time can be financially penalized by the very HMO or PPO which is their employer if they make too many referrals.

However, at the very time that medical insurance companies are attempting to limit your choices, there appears to be a new frontier arising in both health and medicine. This new frontier is the idea that we are responsible for our own bodies and our own health. Alternative medicine appears to have taken a very strong hold on the thinking of Americans, millions of whom are returning to ancient healing traditions in their uneasiness with modern techniques.

The National Institutes of Health have funded a new Office of Alternative Medicine, to explore those alternative medicines Americans are seeking, apparently in droves, as they become dissatisfied with the cost-limiting, high-tech, mechanical, pill-popping ways of modern medicine.

It is possible, as your health improves and your sinuses allow you to feel better as they heal, that you might want to explore for yourself some of these alternatives. However, it is important to be an informed consumer. These alternative medical practices can range from those with long traditions of careful study and exploration to those that are just plain nonsense. Less risky than drugs and surgery, in general, these alternative treatments can be wasteful of your time and money. If you like, you might want to take a look, see if they can be helpful to you. Such a journey can widen your horizons, enlarge your knowledge and help you start on a path toward a healthier life-style.

Holistic Medicine

The practitioner of holistic medicine believes in looking at the causes of disease rather than focusing on the disease, and treating the symptoms presented. A holistic physician wants to restore balance and harmony to the person. The words "health" and "heal" are derived from the Anglo-Saxon word *haelen* which means "to make whole."

The American Holistic Medical Association defines holistic medicine as "a philosophy of medical care which emphasizes personal responsibility and fosters a cooperative doctor/patient relationship." When you go to a physician (or allopath, osteopath, naturopath, chiropractor, dentist or other practitioner of holistic medicine) you will find that you are going to be involved in more than a ten to fifteen minute office visit, a prescription for an antibiotic, and a bill to submit to your insurance company. You should find you will be counseled in life-style choices and methods of self-care.

The American Holistic Medical Association has adopted the following principles of medical practice, and practitioners are expected to adhere to them in their diagnosis and treatment of patients:

1. Embrace a variety of safe, effective options in diagnosis and treatment, including

    a. education for life-style changes and self-care;

    b. complementary approaches; and

    c. conventional drugs and surgery

2. Search for the underlying causes of disease in preference to treating symptoms only.

3. Expend as much effort in establishing what kind of patient has a disease as in establishing what kind of disease a patient has.

4. Treat patients as unique individuals rather than as members of a disease category.

5. Use life-style modifications in preference to drugs and surgery as initial therapeutic options, when possible.

6. Evoke the patient's own innate healing capabilities as the most cost-effective approach. Prevention is preferable to treatment.

7. View the illness as a manifestation of a dysfunction of the whole person, not as an isolated event.

8. Encourage patient autonomy rather than physician-imposed decisions.

9. Consider the needs, desires, awareness and insight of the patient.

10. Know that the quality of the relationship established between physician and patient is a major determinant of healing outcomes.

11. Influence patients by self-example.

12. Acknowledge that illness, pain and the dying process can be learning opportunities for both patients and physicians.

13. Encourage patients to evoke the healing power of love, hope, humor and enthusiasm and to release the toxic consequences of hostility, shame, greed, depression and prolonged fear, anger, or grief.

14. Strive to adopt an attitude of unconditional love for patients, themselves and other practitioners.

15. Acknowledge that optimal health is much more than the absence of sickness; that it the conscious pursuit of the highest qualities of spiritual, mental, emotional, physical, environmental, and social aspects of the human experience.

We have become a nation of fast food, fast information, more and more rapidly performing computers. We want the quickest, the most effortless way of everything, including health and wellness. Science and technology have done a wonderful job of providing us with much of this speed, with amazing machinery that will keep us alive after our bodies have broken down—often the result of our own lack of self-care in our pursuit of careers, fun, more and better "things," and higher and higher incomes. No one should be faulted for wanting a better life, a better home, more education and the good things in life for ourselves and our children. However, it is apparent many of us have paid a very high price for this so-called better life.

In seeking a holistic practitioner, you will not find a quick fix to your sinusitis. Instead, you will find that you may be asked to make life-style changes, to eat differently, exercise, slow down, examine your relationships and the stressors in your life. Ultimately, you will become your own healer, which requires time, effort, and patience, and a commitment to a willingness to change.

Holistic medicine has been called mind/body medicine, and research has confirmed that our thoughts, beliefs, attitudes, emotions and relationships can either strengthen or weaken the immune system. If you are willing to commit yourself to holistic healing you will ultimately become a practitioner of preventive medicine—avoiding abusing your body and mind, and creating an environment in which you can stay well.

Biofeedback

Stress is a large factor in continued ill health. Learning to relax is an important step in improving overall wellness. Biofeedback is a simple way to learn how to relax. It can be enjoyable and is usually successful. Biofeedback is a relaxation technique: the equipment amplifies the responses you already have until they become perceptible and therefore more controllable. Patients learn to raise the temperature of their hands, and by so doing relax the whole sympathetic nervous system, which controls many involuntary functions. It is especially useful in those conditions with a high stress component, such as migraine headaches.

This technique teaches you what it feels like to be relaxed on the inside, and then you are taught how to re-create that feeling on command and make it a part of your daily living. It is a good technique for those who find meditation too abstract a concept, who prefer something more scientific and yet need help in learning to relax.

If you have found that your sinusitis is worse when you are stressed, biofeedback can be a quick method to discovering how to respond to your stress before you are overwhelmed by it and on your way to another sinus attack.

Yoga

Yoga is one of six orthodox systems of Indian philosophy. Hatha yoga, the one Westerners are most familiar with, is a system of stretching, breathing and exercising that many find helpful. For those whose lives are constantly under strain and whose schedules demand top physical and mental fitness, the practice of yoga will discipline the body, the mind and the spirit and provide a relaxation that is most beneficial.

Feeling relaxed and not tense is always beneficial to health, not just to the health of the sinuses. Many individuals who cannot find the time to participate in other kinds of exercise find the slow movements and deep breathing of yoga are excellent for improving the health of the sinuses.

Hypnotherapy

Hypnosis is one of the oldest and most effective psychological interventions available. Essentially, all hypnosis is self-hypnosis, and it instills a sense of control which can be effective.

Hypnotherapy uses the mind/body connection to encourage a trancelike state, during which you will be in a state of heightened suggestibility. In this state, verbal suggestions are able to pass from the mind to the nervous system, influencing the body in ways that seem ordinarily impossible.

A referral to a licensed hypnotherapist can produce excellent results in those who have difficulty in relaxing and letting go of tensions, or whose negative thinking continues to hold them back from changing their attitude about their illness and prevents further healing.

After some training, you are given the tools to use on your own for entering a state of self-hypnosis readily and easily; then you can proceed to use them to control the condition of your sinuses and your pain and discomfort.

Cognitive Therapy

Albert Ellis pioneered this type of psychotherapy which stresses thinking—examining your ideas, beliefs, assumptions and interpretations of the behavior of others.

Cognitive therapists teach you how to critically evaluate your own thinking, rather than adhering to the standards and norms of the outside world. This concept is based on the idea that if you change what you think, you can change the way you feel.

Psychotherapy can be an important method of improving your health. In a study at UCLA School of Medicine involving cancer patients, it was found that those who had psychotherapy had great positive changes in their immune systems.

If you find you are constantly blaming others or your environment or evaluating your life situation negatively, this type of therapy may be beneficial in decreasing the frequency of your common colds, which lead to further sinus problems.

Guided Imagery and Visualization

This form of therapy is beneficial for those who have the ability to visualize and who can be led to think positively about their condition. A professional should be used at first to teach the methods to be sure that you are performing them correctly. Guided imagery and visualization can enhance the effectiveness of other treatments.

Dr. Andrew Weil, in his book *Spontaneous Healing*, says that he believes that no disease process is beyond the reaches of these techniques.

Guided imagery provides a sense of control, engenders a state of relaxation and diverts attention from the pain and discomfort.

With an instructor, the individual is helped to visualize a peaceful, relatively unchanging scene and is encouraged to use the senses of sound, sight, touch, smell and taste to make an image that is as vivid as possible. In this very safe environment the person works on visualizing the sinuses healing, the infection growing smaller and smaller until it disappears entirely.

When our eyes are open, we are drawn to scenes that we perceive outside of ourselves. When our eyes are closed and there is silence, images and thoughts come to us about our inner state. Dreams, daydreams, and fantasies are examples of how our mind pictures what we think and feel.

Guided imagery can have three basic valuable uses:

> Becoming more receptive: to help become more aware of feelings, dissatisfactions, tensions and images that are affecting body functioning.

> Healing: to help erase bacteria or viruses, build new cells to replace damaged ones, make sore areas more comfortable, tense areas relaxed, bring blood to areas that need nutrients or cleansing, make moist areas dry or dry areas moist, bring energy to fatigued areas and enhance general wellness.

> Problem solving: to consult your own intuitive source of wisdom in a structured way or break down barriers to clear thinking.

Body relaxation facilitates the flow of internal messages, so when guided imagery is used it is helpful to first assist the person to a relaxed state. These internal messages can be negative and disturbing, or relaxed and health-producing. With training, you can focus on developing positive, healing images.

If you are an individual with a creative mind, able to visualize readily, you might find that creative visualization will work very rapidly for you—you might enjoy it as a form of therapy that is suited to your creative mind—and your sinuses may thank you.

Osteopathic Medicine

Osteopathic physicians (D.O.s) are, in some ways, very similar to the medical doctors (M.D.s) of today. They go to school as long, study many of the same courses and train in the same residencies upon graduation. They can prescribe medicine and perform surgery—but their orientation to disease is different. *Osteo* from the Latin root of "bone" and *patheia* from the Greek for "passion" or "suffering": osteopathic medical schools teach a holistic philosophy and a hands-on approach to diagnosis and treatment based on the interrelationship of structure (the skeleton of the body, its "bones") and their function. They believe that the human body is in nature and function designed to operate as a harmonious, perfect whole, and that disease in one part affects all other parts.

The osteopath will manipulate the soft tissues (ligaments/facia), the bones of the cranium (the skull), and the muscles. For the head, nose, sinuses and the lungs, these techniques can be very beneficial. Other osteopathic techniques, such as release of the facia and lymphatic drainage, performed at the area of the ribs and the sternum, have been reported to be effective in the treatment of asthma and bronchitis.

Chiropractic

Chiropractic is the manipulation of the spine and is helpful for conditions with acute musculoskeletal pain, tension headaches and for recovery from trauma, such as pressure on the sciatic nerve in the lower back. It is doubtful if it is of much help for sinusitis.

Naturopathic Medicine

Naturopathic physicians (N.D.s) specialize in natural medicine. They are trained at very specialized four-year medical colleges and are educated in the conventional medical sciences. The difference lies in the treatment of disease. Their treatments are drawn from clinical nutrition, herbal and botanical medicine, homeopathy, traditional Chinese medicine, exercise therapy, acupuncture and hydrotherapy. A naturopath might combine several of these treatments or specialize in a specific area.

Naturopathy is based on the concept that the body is self-healing. The effort of this physician is to enhance the body's own immune system through non-invasive measures.

There are only two naturopathic medical colleges in the U.S. today, as they declined with the advent of pharmaceuticals and the belief early in this century that drugs could cure everything. However, as more and more people have been returning to alternative medicine, there appears to be a renewed interest in this type of medicine.

For those interested in being responsible for their own health, for improving the health of their sinuses through more natural means, and who wish to find a physician who will aid them in making life-style changes through improved nutrition and the use of botanical medicine, a naturopath might be a good choice.

Meditation

Meditation is something that many of us consider almost impossible to do. We are so busy running, hurrying, entertaining ourselves constantly with television or other activities that we have almost forgotten how to do this.

There is really nothing mysterious about meditation. It is simply sitting quietly and focusing on some one thing, usually your own breathing. It slows you down and allows you to inhale more oxygen while it keeps you focused on the present, rather than worrying about the past or the future.

Most stress management programs now include a period of meditation practice: it is used in hospital programs to lower blood pressure, and slow the heart rate of those in cardiac care and chronic pain clinics.

Busy people, those always on the run, seem to resist any kind of slowing-down type therapy. They are probably just the ones who need this type of therapy the most. Sometimes a commitment to the half-hour or so that such a practice requires is doubly beneficial to this kind of busy person in conquering stress and bringing healing blood flow to the sinuses.

For those interested in more information on meditation, how to do it and how to use it in your everyday life, there are a number of useful books, such as *Meditation in Everyday Life* by Jon Kabat-Zinn and *How to Meditate* by Lawrence LeShan.

Body Work

Body work is generally considered massage therapy, and it can be very useful in relaxing tight muscles and reducing stress. There are a variety of very specific body work theories, and anyone interested in them can usually find a practitioner through the yellow pages, traditional massage therapists, gyms or health food stores.

Because these body work therapies are excellent in reducing stress, they can be useful for busy people who find they frequently have tight muscles throughout the body, with tension headaches caused by tight neck muscles constricting blood flow to the head.

Feldenkrais is a system of movements, floor exercises and body work designed to retrain the central nervous system to help it find new pathways around areas of blockage. This system is innovative, gentle and often much more helpful than standard physical therapy.

Rolfing is a more invasive form of massage. It is directed at restructuring the musculoskeletal system by working on patterns of tension held in deep tissue. The therapist applies very firm pressure to different areas of the body, which can be quiet painful. Practitioners believe they are releasing repressed emotions which have translated into unrelenting tension in the muscles.

Shiatsu is a traditional healing form from Japan. The therapist uses firm finger pressure applied to specific points on the body to increase the circulation of vital energy. In some ways, this is similar to acupressure, but the pressure is much stronger and can be uncomfortable.

Trager is the least invasive of the body works. It uses gentle rocking and bouncing motions to induce a state of deep relaxation. It is used to help facilitate the nervous system's communication with muscles, and is helpful for individuals who, for a variety of physical reasons, cannot tolerate more strenuous massage or pressure.

Peace of Mind

Many people are unaware of the mind/body connection in disease; if we ever give it any thought, our personal experience will tell us that our mind and body are connected. We experience "self" as a combination of both the physical and mental. Sometimes we may be more aware of our body (i.e., pain) and at other times our mind (i.e., in solving a mathematical problem), but we cannot experience one without the other. We cannot experience pain without consciousness, and we cannot experience mental states without the anatomic and physiologic functioning of a brain. A simple example of proof of this fact is that you cannot tickle yourself. The response depends on more than mere touch; certain mental interactions are necessary to make a touch a tickle.

The way you think has a profound impact on your life. Everything you do is a result of your thinking. How you spend your leisure time, what you do for a living, your values and goals, the concepts you have of what family means, the friends you choose, what you are willing to accept as the quality of your life.

Every human being has psychological needs. Everyone needs to give and receive love; everyone needs to feel they belong and that they are significant; everyone needs to feel secure; everyone needs to explore and learn; and everyone needs to create something that adds meaning to their lives. Children learn to imitate adults in the satisfaction of these needs. Through a process of trial and error, adults taught you what you had to do to receive love and what they would accept from you in return as love. You were taught what behavior was acceptable so that you would be included in the family unit, and what you could do to receive recognition, both positive and negative. You were taught how far you could go in exploring new thoughts or actions, and what and how to learn. You were taught what you could create and how you could create it. You were disciplined or not, and through the experience of the consequences of your actions—through trial and error—your needs were met in a negative or positive way.

The result of all that is that you have a self-image and a particular way of responding and acting. All of us have an internal dialogue, we are talking to ourselves all day long, and what we say to ourselves has a great deal to do with our state of mental health. If these messages are generally self-critical, filled with "I should have" or "I wish I hadn't," they will have a negative impact on health, both physical and mental.

Identifying and understanding the stresses you are subjected to, and which you subject yourself to from your internal dialogue, must be an integral part of any successful therapy. Unless you can adapt successfully to life's stresses, the pursuit of health may be a long and trying process.

Faith and Healing

More and more medical schools are adding courses on holistic and alternative medicine with titles like "Caring for the Soul."

This change reflects a yearning among patients of today for a more personal, more spiritual approach to health and healing. This is obviously a growing disenchantment with one of the greatest achievements of the 20th century: high-tech medicine. As we are all aware, Western medicine is at its best in a crisis—battling acute infection, repairing the complex wounds of high speed transportation accidents, gunshot wounds, replacing organs. But increasingly, all prosperous societies suffer from chronic illnesses, such as high blood pressure, back problems, cardiovascular disease, arthritis and acute problems that frequently become chronic. In most of these, as in sinusitis, stress and life-style play a part.

Dr. Herbert Benson, president of the Mind/ Body Medical Institution of Boston's Deaconess

Hospital and Harvard Medical School, says, "Anywhere from sixty to ninety percent of visits to doctors are in the mind-body, stress related realm."

There is a shift among many practitioners today toward acceptance of the concept that there may be more to health than blood-cell counts and EKGs; more to healing than pills and surgery.

In a ground-breaking study conducted by Dr. Elisabeth Targ, clinical director of psychosocial oncology research at California Pacific Medical Center in San Francisco, twenty faith healers used prayer to attempt to heal twenty severely ill AIDS patients. Targ describes the results as sufficiently encouraging to warrant a larger follow-up study.

Alienated patients, tired of the endless high-tech procedures of modern medicine, are now spending $30 billion a year in the offices of alternative therapists and faith healers. Millions more are spent on bestselling books and tapes by New Age doctors such as Deepak Chopra, who has become a one-man health industry.

A 1955 study at Dartmouth-Hitchcock Medical Center found that one of the best predictors of survival among several heart surgery patients was the degree to which they said they drew comfort and strength from religious faith. Those who did not had more than three times the death rate of those who did.

A survey of 30 years research on blood pressure by Dr. David Larson at National Institute for Healthcare Research, a privately funded institute, found that churchgoers have 5 mm lower blood pressure than non-churchgoers.

A 1996 National Institute on Aging study of 4,000 elderly persons living at home in North Carolina found those who attended religious services were physically healthier and less depressed than those who did not attend.

In another study of thirty female patients recovering from hip fractures, those who regarded God as a source of strength and comfort and who attended religious services were able to walk farther upon discharge and had lower rates of depression than those with little faith.

Numerous other studies have found lowered rates of depression and anxiety-related illnesses among the religiously committed.

Dr. Benson, whose bestselling book *The Relaxation Response* described success in battling stress-related illnesses by a simple form of meditation believes that meditation (or prayer) operate along the same biochemical pathways as the relaxation response. The act of focusing the mind on a single sound or image brings about a set of physiological changes that are the opposite of the "fight-or-flight" response. Meditation affects epinephrine and other corticosteroid messengers—the stress hormones—which leads to lower blood pressure, more relaxed heart and respiration rates, as well as other physiological benefits.

Recent research demonstrates these stress hormones also have a direct impact on the body's immunological defenses against disease. Dr. David Felton, chairman of the Department of Neurobiology at the University of Rochester, says: "Anything involved with meditation and controlling the state of mind that alters hormone activity has the potential to have an impact on the immune system."

Even more interesting is the fact that years of research have shown that if a patient truly believes a therapy is useful—voodoo, witch doctors beating on drums, whatever their culture has said is curative—that belief has the power to heal.

Does this imply to be truly cured you have to be religious? Certainly not. It points to being or behaving in a way that includes some quiet time for reflection, for thinking, for meditation, for bringing together whatever forces are within yourself to bear on healing your ailing tissue. The whole person, not just the body or the mind, but the part that includes the spiritual inner person: whatever the beliefs held, in some traditional organized religion or some type of New Age life-force in the abstract, belief seems to be necessary to give strength, focus, and quiet time to help you heal yourself.

For those who want to explore this further, it may not be necessary to understand how prayer or meditation works to put it to good use in aiding in the healing of your sinuses.

Further reading might include, *Prayer is Good Medicine* by Larry Dossey, a Santa Fe internist; *You Can Heal Your Life* by Louise Hay; John Kabat-Zinn's *Full Catastrophe Living* or *Spontaneous Healing* by Andre Weil. These are just a few of the books updating some of the differing philosophies on healing, and simplifying the understanding of visualization techniques for meditation and prayer so they can be applied to your health.

Acupressure and Acupuncture

Acupressure and acupuncture are ancient forms of healing. Acupressure encompasses *shiatsu,* a Japanese form of rhythmically applied pressure; *do-in,* an Oriental self-care practice that includes movement, stretching, and invigorating self-massage techniques; *tui na,* a Chinese form of massage designed to release muscle tension; and *acu-yoga,* an ancient Asian healing practice that combines yoga poses, stretching, breathing, and meditation, using the whole body to simulate acupressure points.

Acupressurists press and stimulate key energy points on the body to affect the flow of vital energy within the person. This in turn stimulates the body's ability to heal itself.

The location of the key points are based on the Eastern concept of the body as an energy vessel. From the point of view of the traditional healers of China, India, and Japan, the body contains more than a dozen specific energy channels, or meridians, that direct the flow of energy. The meridians are the same on both sides of the body and are named for the organ systems that the channels are associated with, such as the gall bladder or the kidney. From the Oriental perspective, the meridian system is not merely hidden, blood-vessel-like channels: it is an intricate set of relationships and communications between organs, systems, and senses.

The life energy that is said to flow in these channels is called *qi* (or chi) by the Chinese, *ki* by the Japanese, and *prana* by the people of India. The life energy runs smoothly and harmoniously in the body of a person who is active and healthy, but is said to be blocked or deficient in a person who suffers from an illness or injury.

Practitioners of traditional Oriental medicine have developed a number of techniques to stimulate or balance the flow of energy. The energy model is the basis of *acupuncture*, in which slim needles are inserted into the skin at special points, and *moxibustion*, in which heat is applied to the skin. Since acupressure practitioners press on the body's vital energy points primarily with the fingers and hands, acupressure is the simplest and easiest-to-use method for harmonizing the body's life energies and balancing the flow of energy. Acupressure techniques are also the most practical for first-aid and self-care techniques.

These are key acupressure points for sinus and breathing difficulties. Do them once a day.

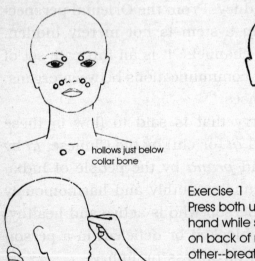

o o hollows just below collar bone

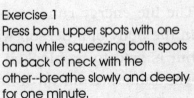

Exercise 1
Press both upper spots with one hand while squeezing both spots on back of neck with the other--breathe slowly and deeply for one minute.

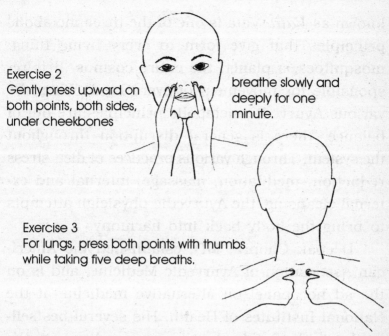

Exercise 2
Gently press upward on both points, both sides, under cheekbones

breathe slowly and deeply for one minute.

Exercise 3
For lungs, press both points with thumbs while taking five deep breaths.

Another simple technique for sinus is to press on the roof of your mouth with your thumb or with a teaspoon for several seconds. Repeat until you feel some relief.

Ayurveda

Ayurveda is considered the traditional medicine of India. It comes from the Sanskrit words, *Ayus,* or "life" and *Veda,* meaning "science" or "knowledge" There is a deep spiritual basis for Ayurveda: the promotion of longevity without limit, and the belief that life is essentially immortal.

According to this traditional medicine, the life energy is channeled throughout the body by a "wind" known as *Vata.* Vata is one of the three metabolic principles that give form to every living thing: mosquitoes, a planet, the entire cosmos. It is responsible for movement of every kind. When the various Ayurvedic metabolic principles are out of balance, there is general disruption throughout the system. Through various practices of diet, stress reduction, meditation, massage, internal and external cleansing, the Ayurvedic physician attempts to bring the body back into harmony.

Deepak Chopra, MD, established the American Association of Ayurvedic Medicine, and is on the ad hoc panel on alternative medicine at the National Institutes of Health. His several bestselling books have introduced a new audience to the concepts of this ancient healing art, and indicate the general dissatisfaction many Americans have with the high-tech way of modern medicine.

For those interested in reading more about this 5,000-year-old system of Ayurveda, *Perfect Health* and *Ageless Body, Timeless Mind* by Dr. Chopra make the concept and its practices—for reestablishing the body's natural balance and for strengthening the mind/body connection—easily understood by the Western reader.

Traditional Chinese Medicine

Traditional Chinese medicine is one of the oldest

systems known. Dating back almost five thousand years, it uses the history and observation of the entire body (particularly the tongue), palpation and pulse diagnosis (a technique which is it said takes almost ten years to learn properly).

Chinese physicians believe that a certain process must take place before the body develops a problem or disease, and they look for this in a pattern of bodily disharmony. Ill health is seen as an imbalance between the body's nutritive substances, known as *yin,* and the functional activity of the body, known as *yang.* This imbalance can cause a disruption of the flow of the vital energy that circulates through pathways in the body.

Treatment usually includes dietary changes, massage, medicinal teas and other preparations made primarily from herbs, acupuncture and moxibustion (the burning of herbs at acupuncture points). Because this system treats the whole person and not just symptoms, there appears to be a conjoining of the mind, body, emotions, spirit and environment in this treatment system.

Many Chinese remedies appear to have significant therapeutic value and are worth trying for a wide range of allergies, infections and chronic conditions, including asthma, chronic sinusitis and bronchitis and other states of immune deficiency.

The World Health Organization has published a list of over fifty conditions successfully treated with Chinese medicine. Included in this list are sinusitis, asthma, headaches and allergies.

Herbalism

Plants are the most widely used tool there is in natural medicine. The tradition of using leaves, roots, seeds, and other parts of a plant as medicine goes back tens of thousands of years.

Scientists have been studying how different cultures throughout the world have been using plant remedies for a variety of medicinal effects. Various herbs have been found to relieve pain, stop or induce vomiting, reduce inflammation, lower a fever, stimulate the bowels, soothe nerves, promote relaxation and sleep, and invigorate and strengthen the whole body.

Herbal companies have developed standardized commercial extracts, and those who favor such standardization contend that research has identified the important active factors; such extracts make it easier for average individuals to go into a health food store and find the herb they want without having to grow their own or know about soil conditions, weather, harvesting and drying techniques. It is helpful to get some assistance in the use of herbs because they come in a variety of forms and are used in a variety of ways: teas, infusions, decoctions, tinctures, tablets, capsules and lozenges. There are a number of excellent herbal books available which should aid in the identification and use of herbs.

Herbs are generally safe and nontoxic but should be used with knowledge and caution. No responsible herbalist ever says that all herbs are safe. They are usually much safer than synthetic drugs, but they are complex mixtures of chemical compounds that can heal, change different bodily processes and sometimes cause side effects, particularly when overused or used inappropriately.

Below are some examples of herbs that are beneficial for specific conditions:

Allergy: nettles, echinacea, red clover, eyebright, golden seal, ephedra, elder.

Anticatarrhal: elder, golden seal, myrrh, sandalwood, hyssop.

Antifungal: garlic, pau d'arco, propolis, Candida, cinnamon, black walnut.

Anti-inflammatory: oak bark, passion flower, white willow, plantain, meadowsweet, devils claw.

Antimicrobial: myrrh, echinacea, garlic, wild indigo, mullein, thyme.

Antiseptic: black walnut, oak bark, thyme, peppermint, propolis, sage, myrrh, wild indigo.

Anti-viral: St. John's wort, echinacea, garlic, astragalus.

Asthma: mullein, coltsfoot, golden seal, ma huang, lobelia, ginkgo biloba, horehound, licorice, elecampane, blessed thistle, wild cherry, blue cohosh.

Bronchial support: schizandra, mullein, coltsfoot, fenugreek, horehound, hyssop, licorice, pleurisy root, elecampane, thyme, myrrh, golden seal.

Colds/flu: echinacea, pleurisy root, catnip, peppermint, boneset, elder.

Cough: wild cherry bark, licorice, slippery elm, coltsfoot, horehound.

Ear ache: mullein oil, garlic, sage.

Expectorant: elcampane, fenugreek, plantain, thyme, horehound, hyssop, licorice, sage, mullein, garlic.

Fever: sage, thyme, echinacea, white willow, nettles, blue vervian, wild indigo, yarrow.

Hayfever: nettles, echinacea.

Immune support: astragalus, reishi, nettles, shitake, schizandra, echinacea, propolis, garlic, pau d'arco, chaparral.

Pain: hops, white willow, valerian.

Recovery tonics: gota kola, ginseng, nettles, fo-ti, passion flower, astrgalus, schizandra.

Respiratory: horehound, mullein, myrrh, astragalus, golden seal, elecampane.

Rhinitis: nettles, echinacea, astragalus.

Sore throat: fennel, ginger, peppermint, chamomile.

If you wish to put together a first-aid kit of the most basic and essential herbs for sinusitis to have in your home, it should include:

calendula
chamomile
comfrey
echinacea
ephedra
goldenseal
pau d'arco
plantain
slippery elm
white willow

All herbs may have contraindications—such as not to be used during pregnancy, or for individuals with other medical conditions, such as high blood pressure or heart disease. A qualified holistic herbalist, a holistic practitioner or your family physician should be consulted prior to using any herbs.

Homeopathy

Homeopathy is derived from the Greek words *homoio* meaning "similar" and *pathos*, for "disease" or "suffering." The German physician Samuel

Hahnemann discovered in the mid-1800s that certain diseases were cured by giving minute doses of drugs that in a healthy person would produce symptoms like those of the disease. He called this idea "like cures like" or "the law of similars."

His ideas were fundamentally opposite to the theory of allopathy, from the Greek *allos* which means "other" and is the basis for the thinking of conventional medicine. His theory was that the best treatment of disease was gentle and simple, and he began to experiment with very tiny doses of herbs, minerals and other substances.

Hahnemann maintained the presence of very small amounts of one of his remedies in the body stimulated the body's ability to fight off the disease. He believed that symptoms are as much a part of the healing process as they are of disease. He felt when you suppressed symptoms it only drove the disease deeper into the body where it would reoccur, manifesting itself in a more serious condition. He wanted to give the body no more than a little push in the right direction, to prime its pump so to speak, to bring forth its own natural healing powers. Through experimentation, Hahnemann found extremely dilute solutions were effective, but did not cause unwanted side effects.

Present day homeopaths use smaller and smaller amounts of a variety of substances, primarily derived from plants. Traditional modern physicians contend the minute amounts of the active substances in these diluted remedies cannot possibly have any physical effects on the body. Homeopaths argue that vaccinations, in which a very minute amount of the pathogen produces immunity by causing the body to produce antigens (such as in the immunizations against smallpox and polio) have proven that this method is effective.

They further state that certain essential trace vitamins and minerals are absorbed and utilized by the body in infinitesimal quantities, yet their absence determines health or illness. They cite the fact that 50 to 100 millionths of a gram of the thyroid hormone is manufactured by the body each day, resulting in a concentration in the normal blood of one part per 10,000 million parts of blood plasma. Yet if this amount is missing, faulty metabolism and illness result.

Homeopathy goes one step further. It is thought that there is a mysterious, nonphysical nature to these remedies. That they contain "the essence of the substance, its resonance, its energy." This essence is thought to interact with the life force of the individual; in a manner similar to that of the *qi* of the Oriental systems of medicine.

Homeopathic remedies are regulated by the U.S. Food and Drug Administration (FDA), and it has taken the position that these homeopathic remedies are safe and nontoxic.

It is also well known that the Royal Family of England faithfully use homeopathy and homeopathic physicians, and have done so all their lives.

The homeopathic physician prescribes very minute particles—the essence of the extract—in their preparations. For example, a practitioner might prescribe extract of belladonna, derived from the poisonous plant deadly nightshade *(Atropa belladonna)*, to treat fever or flu because it causes fever, flushing, delirium and other flu-like symptoms when ingested in large amounts. However, the amount of belladonna contained in a homeopathic treatment is minute. That is because they are formulated according to Dr. Hahnemann's "law of infinitesimals," which states that the smaller the dose, the more potent the cure. Dr. Hahnemann believed that vigorously shaking the solution each time it was diluted "potentialized" it, leaving behind a "spirit-like" essence that cures by activating the body's "vital force." One of the largest selling homeopathic drugs is Oscillococcinum, a cold and flu remedy made from the heart and liver of wild Barbary ducks—which carry flu virus.

Edward Chapman, president of the American Institute of Homeopathy believes that the use of homeopathic remedies, "changes the underlying pattern of the immune system," giving the body only a very tiny slight boost in the direction it needs to heal itself.

These preparations are available, in both tablet and liquid form, over-the-counter. A chart is provided for the purchaser to look up existing symptoms to find the appropriate medicine. For those interested in homeopathy, it is probably best to consult a homeopathic physician for treatment.

Your first aid kit for homeopathic remedies for your sinuses might include:

acomte

cepis

arsenicum

calendula

hupericum

ledum

rhus tox

ruta

Flower Essences

Edward Bach, a British homeopath and pathologist, began in the 1930s to explore the healing secrets of wildflower blossoms.

The Flower essences are liquid remedies made from wildflower blossoms. These formulations do not address specific physical illnesses but moods, attitudes, and emotions such as fear, anxiety and restlessness. As in homeopathy, flower essence practice is a form of subtle energy medicine. They work on the emotional state of the individual. Their aim is to transform the negative attitudes associated with the disease into positive ones. This, in turn, allows the body's own physical system to fight that disease and its associated stress. The remedies are said to work on a vibrational rather than biochemical basis. The flowers are prescribed to act as a gentle catalyst, promoting the body to heal itself.

The Bach Flower Essences, a standard group of thirty-eight flower essences, is known worldwide and these medications are sold by the millions of bottles yearly.

The flower essences are taken by adding 2 to 4 drops of the chosen essence to a glass of water or juice, to be sipped at intervals. The essence selected is based on a self-questionnaire that will guide you in your selection based on how you are feeling at the moment. Any health food store can provide a useful summary of the essences, or you might want to read the book *Bach Flower Essences for the Family* or *Bach Flower Remedies Step by Step*

The flower essence for your sinus first aid kit is Rescue remedy. Rescue remedy is composed of five of the essences and can be taken for a wide variety of situations. It can be taken any time the individual feels stressed to aid in the return to a positive state of mind.

Aromatherapy and the Use of Essential Oils

Aromatherapists use essential oils derived from the leaves, barks, roots, flowers, resins, and seeds of plants to assist in the recovery from physical and psychological problems.

Typically the oils are inhaled for respiratory problems and applied topically or added to the bath for skin and muscle problems.

A number of ancient civilizations used aromatic plants, gums, and oils in their cooking, cosmetics, or spiritual practices. The Babylonians, the Chinese and the Egyptians learned how to distill plants to obtain these essential oils. The Egyptians used gums and oils of cedar and myrrh in the mummification process in an effort to retard the decay of the physical body. Odors in the form of incense have been used for centuries in a variety of spiritual practices, and essential oils and herbs were an integral part of Western medicine until the advent of scientific chemistry and synthetic drug development in the last century.

It is well known that our sense of smell has a close connection to mood, emotions and sexual desire. These connections have long been recognized by the perfume industry, a major producer and buyer of essential oils until the advent of synthetic fragrances.

Scientists have isolated hundreds of components in just one essential oil, so it would not be surprising to think that they might have myriad effects on our emotions.

Essential oils are volatile, quickly evaporating and, properly used, should have no side effects. Measured by the drop, most essential oils are diluted before being applied to the body.

If the emotions and psychological health are closely tied to sinus infections, as is thought by a number of homeopathic physicians, then the use of essential oils in aiding relaxation from the stresses of life, in improving moods and increasing your ability to decrease the tensions in the muscles, could be a beneficial practice at the end of a difficult day.

Your first-aid kit of essential oils for your sinusitis would include:

chamomile—a natural tranquilizer and anti-inflammatory

eucalyptus—combats coughs and colds

lavender—a stimulant to the immune system and a natural antibiotic

peppermint—an aid to the respiratory system and ideal for treating headaches

There are several methods for using oils. One of the simplest is to add oils to a pan of boiling water and inhale the vapors. Or use the oil in a relaxing bath, or use an aromatic diffuser that uses only a few drops of the oil and disperses the healing droplets throughout the room in a fine mist.

Professional aromatherapists combine essential oils with massage therapy. These oils are highly volatile, which means they are absorbed directly into the bloodstream through the skin and rush to those parts of the body where they are needed the most.

Reflexology

Reflexology is a science that believes that there are areas of the feet and hands that correspond to all the glands, organs and parts of the body. The practitioner uses the thumb and fingers to exert pressure and then massage the reflex areas of the feet that correspond to those of the body. This pressure is done to relieve stress and tension, improve blood supply and promote the unblocking of nerve impulses in an effort to aid the body to achieve a balanced state of health.

Reflexologists' beliefs grew out of the theories and techniques of acupuncture and acupressure. This system attempts to strengthen and balance the life energy that is thought to flow in meridians or zones of the body. Practitioners specify ten energy zones that run the length of the body from head to toe—five on each side of the body ending in each foot and running down the arms into the tips of the fingers. These zones run through the body also, and all the organs and body parts lie along one or more of these energy zones. By stimulating or working any zone in the foot it is thought this pressure will affect the entire zone throughout the body. It is a natural, non-invasive specialty which has been found to be effective as a treatment for a number of ailments. Very possibly the massage of the foot induces a state of relaxation, thus reducing stresses in the body. Obviously, by massage, circulation can be improved, energy levels increased, mood can be heightened.

The sinus points are the ends of the fingers and toes, from the crease to the tips, front and back. Gently squeeze each one, with a slight circular rubbing motion, for about one minute each. The lungs correspond to the pads on the palms and soles just below the fingers and toes.

If you are interested in exploring reflexology as a part of a holistic health program, you might want to visit a reflexologist first, to have an expert show you the pressure points, how much pressure to apply and for how long. Then try stimulating these points daily and see if it has any effect on your sinuses.

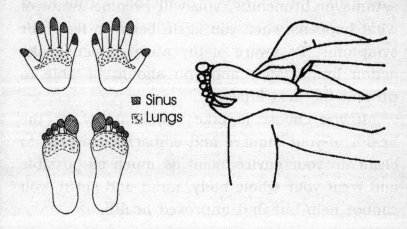

☒ Sinus
☒ Lungs

Massage firmly at the bases of your four digits on both hands and feet. If your breathing improves, then massage the bases of your thumbs and big toes. Can be repeated as often as desired.

Press your thumbs firmly on both sides of your nose and hold for 30 seconds. Repeat.

All the systems of the respiratory tract—the nose, the sinuses, the lungs, the bronchi and the ears—are interconnected. Anyone interested in protecting any part of this system needs to be aware that you cannot deal with just one alone: they are part of a whole.

As you begin to take charge you will become aware of what makes you feel better and what makes you feel worse. If you find that there are periods when you are free of infection, allergy, or asthma or bronchitis, you will become aware of what happens when you again begin to feel your symptoms. Be aware of the warning signs, take action immediately and you should be able to prevent the next attack.

If you choose to take responsibility for the health of your sinuses and embark on a plan to clean up your environment as much as possible and treat your whole body, mind and spirit, you cannot help but find improved health.

Bibliography

Anderson, Robert A. *Wellness Medicine.* New Canaan, CT: Keats, 1990.

Barinaga, Marcia. "Carbon Monoxide." *Science,* January 15, 1993.

Beardsley, Tim. "Resisting Resistance." *Scientific American,* January 1996.

Benedict, Martha S. "Holistic Approaches to Colds and Flu." *Body Mind Spirit,* February/March 1995.

Benson, Herbert. *The Relaxation Response.* New York: Random House, 1992.

Berkow, Robert, ed. *The Merck Manual.* 16th ed. Rahway, NJ: Mercy & Co., 1992.

Boggs, Peter B. *Sneezing Your Head Off?* New York: Simon and Schuster, 1992.

Brune, Jeffrey. "Lost Horizons." *Discover,* January 1991.

Castleman, Michael. "Tiny Particles, Big Problems." *Sierra,* November/December 1995.

Chopra, Deepak. *Perfect Health.* New York: Harmony, 1991.

———. *Ageless Body, Timeless Mind.* New York: Harmony, 1993.

Clerico, Dean M. and David W. Kennedy. "Chronic Sinusitis: Diagnostic and Treatment Advances." *Hospital Medicine*, July 1994.

Creticos, Peter S., et.al. "Ragweed Immunotherapy in Adult Asthma." *The New England Journal of Medicine*, February 22, 1996.

Couzens, Gerald Secor. "Breathtaking Workouts." *Women's Sport & Fitness*, September 1991.

Darrow, Paula. "The Best Allergy Treatments." *American Health*. March 1995.

Dieterich, Robert. "The Body Electric." *The Sciences*, May/June 1995.

Dossey, Larry. *Healing Words.* San Francisco: Harper, 1993.

———. *Prayer is Good Medicine*. San Francisco: Harper, 1996.

Fishein, Richard. "Treating Asthma Without Drugs." *Natural Health*, July/August 1994.

Freifeld, Karen. "By a Nose." *Health,* August 1987.

Gach, Michael Reed. *Accupressure's Potent Points.* Harpers, 1989.

Gloeckner, Carolyn. "Life with Asthma." *Current Health*, April 1989.

Hay, Louise L. *You Can Heal Your Life.* Hay House, 1990.

Hendeles, Leslie, Miles Weinberger, and Lai Wong. "Medical Management of Noninfectious Rhinitis." *American Journal of Hospital Pharmacy*, November 1980.

Horgan, John. "Radon's Risks." *Scientific American*. August 1994.

Hughes, Rebecca. "Ear Fears" *American Health*. December 1991.

Iovine, John. "Electromagnetic Fields and Your Health." *Popular Mechanics,* March 1994.

Ivker, Robert S. *Sinus Survival*. New York: Putnam Books, 1995.

Johnson, Howard M., et.al. "Superantigens in Human Disease." *Scientific American*, April 1992.

Kabat-Zinn, Jon. *Full Catastrophe Living*. Hyperion, 1994.

LeShan, Lawrence. *How to Meditate*. New York: Doubleday, 1992.

Luckmann, Joan and Karen Creason Sorensen. *Medical-Surgical Nursing*. Philadelphia: W.B. Sauders, 1974.

Laliberte, Richard. "Breathing Uneasy." *Health*, September 1990.

Lehman, H. Jane. "Energy-efficiency Labels for Your Home?" *Consumer's Research Magazine*, December 1995.

Lewis, Alan E. and Dallas Clouatre. *Melatonin and the Biological Clock*. Keats, 1996.

Lewis, Ricki. "The Rise of Antibiotic-resistant Infections." *FDA Consumer,* September 1995.

Lichtenstein, Lawrence M. "Allergy and the Immune System." *Scientific American*, September 1993.

Mattill, John I. "More Electricity, Less Pollution." *Technology Review*, May/June 1991.

Miller, Julie Ann. "Gases Carry Messages in Nervous System." *BioScience*, February 1993.

McCafferty, Phil and Sandy Fritz. "Good Machines for Bad Allergies." *Popular Science*, October 1994.

Monroe, Judy. "Antihistamines and Decongestants." *Current Health*, January 1995.

Nesse, Randolph M. and George C. Williams. "Nothing to Sneeze At." *The Sciences*, November/December 1994.

New, Amy Roffmann. "Controlling 'yeast' Infections." *FDA Consumer,* December 1993.

Novitt-Moreno, Anne. "Antibiotics—Miracle Drugs?" *Current Health*, December 1995.

O'Connell, Linda Matys. "Sick Building Syndrome." *E: the Environmental Magazine*, January/ February 1995.

Patlak, Margie. "Children's All-Too-Common Ear Infections." *FDA Consumer,* December/January 1988.

Pennisi, Elizabeth. "Food Allergies Linked to Ear Infections." *Science News*, October 8, 1994.

Radetsky, Peter. "Of Parasites & Pollens." *Discover,* September 1993.

Raloff, Janet. "When Nitrate Reigns." *Science News*, February 11, 1995.

———. "Food Allergy." *Science News*, August 8, 1992.

Rapp, Doris. *Allergies and Your Family*. Buffalo, NY: Practical Allergy, 1990.

Rector-Page, Linda. *Colds & Flu & You*. Sonora, CA: Healthy Healing, 1995.

Russell, A.G., et.al. "Urban Ozone Control and Atmospheric Reactivity of Organic Gases." *Science,* July 28, 1995.

Saltus, Richard. "Antibiotics—Overused & Misunderstood." *American Health,* October 1995.

Schlatter, Thomas. "On the Move with CFCs." *Weatherwise,* October/November 1995.

Seligson, Susan. "The Big Sneeze." *Health,* September 1995.

Service, Robert F. "Antibiotics that Resist Resistance." *Science*, November 3, 1995.

Sullum, Jacob. "Imbalancing Act." *National Review*, January 23, 1995.

Thiemens, Mark H., et.al. "Carbon Dioxide and Oxygen Isotope Anomalies in the Mesosphere and Stratosphere." *Science*, November 10, 1995.

Tortora, Gerard J. and Nicholas P. Anagnostakos. *Principles of Anatomy and Physiology*. Canfield, 1975.

Weil, Andrew. *Spontaneous Healing.* New York: Knopf, 1995.

Wilen, Joan and Lydia Wilen. *Live and Be Well*. Harper, 1992.

Winter, Ruth. *A Consumer's Guide to Medicines in Food*. New York: Crown, 1995.

Wolf, Moondance. *Rainbow Medicine.* New York: Sterling, 1994.

Wunderlich, Ray C. *Natural Alternatives to Antibiotics*. New Canaan, CT: Keats, 1995.

Zamula, Evelyn. "More Than Snuffles." *FDA Consumer*, July/August, 1990.

Index

A

Acid rain 59
Acid/alkaline balance 36
Acquired immunity 34
Acupressure 276
Acupuncture 276, 277
Acute bronchitis 178
Acute irritative bronchitis 110
Acute otitis media 22
Acute sinusitis 43, 88, 119
Adenoids 75
Air pollution
    indoor 60
    outdoor 53
Alcohol 190, 219
Allergen 66
    air borne 73
    avoiding 172
    definition 165
Allergic asthma shots 177
Allergic rhinitis 106
Allergy 66, 214, 282
    asthma 98
    description 165
    food 67, 109
        children, otitis media 27
        elimination diet 70
    parasitic worms 166
    temporary relief of mild 176
Allergy Free Inc. 151
Allergy shots 177
Analgesics 133
Angioedema 45
Anti-inflammatory 282
Anti-viral 283

Antibiotics 121
    immune system 125
Antibodies 32, 33
Anticattarhal 282
Anticholinergic agents 158
Antifungal 282
Antigens 32, 33
Antihistamines 131, 176
    children 131
    enlarged prostate 132
Antimicrobial 283
Antioxidants 200, 201, 205
Antiseptic 283
Antitussives 132
Aromatherapy 242, 289
Aspirin-induced asthma 151
Asthma 92, 141, 283
    allergic form 100
    allergy 98
    aspirin-induced 151
    athletes 146
    bronchial 99
    children and smoke 51
    diagnosis 103, 147
    dosing for optimal benefit 163
    drugs 155
    gas stoves 152
    management 144
    myths 104
    pollution 96
    pregnancy 169
    pulmonary function test 148
    race and 96
    sinusitis 98
    stress 105
    treatment 150

viruses 98
women 95, 152
Asthma attack 100, 105, 141
  severity, classified 103
Asthmatic bronchitis 110
Athletes and asthma 146
Autoallergens 167
Autoimmune diseases 32
Automobile exhaust 112
Ayurveda 278

B

B-adrenergic agents 155
B2-adrenergics 155
Bilateral middle antrostomy 140
Biofeedback 255
Blankets 246
Body work 267
Bronchial asthma 99
Bronchial support 283
Bronchitis 79, 109
  acute 178
  acute irritative 110
  asthmatic 110
  chronic 110, 178, 179
  obstructive, chronic 182
Bronchodilators 159

C

Caffeine 192, 196
Calcium 210
Caldwell-Luc operation 140
Candida albicans 126, 235
Carbon monoxide 54, 55, 117
Cats 107, 228
Cellulitis 45
Children
  antihistamines 131
  asthma
    fat in diet 154
    fish oil in diet 154

sugar in diet 154
smoke 51
bronchitis 56
herbs 207
ear infections 23
food allergy
  otitis media 27
  test 27
mucus production 83
otitis media 26
  antibiotics 29
pain relievers 133
pollution 56
saline irrigation 137
sinusitis 44, 82
swimmer's ear 31
Chiropractic 264
Chronic bronchitis 110, 178, 179
  obstructive 183
Chronic diseases, top ten 92
Chronic sinusitis 43, 90
  diagnosis 85
Cigarette 50
Cilia 10, 50
Cockroaches 228
Cognitive Therapy 260
Cold 37, 38, 49, 193
Cold air 63
Cold/flu 283
Contactants 165, 167
Corticosteroids 156, 158
Cough 80, 283
Cough suppressants 132
Coughing 243
Croolyn sodium 158
Croup 98
Cyst 76

D

Dairy products 210
Dander 107

Decongestant nasal sprays 129
Decongestants 128, 176
Deviated septum 75
Diet 209
Dizziness 81
Dogs 228
Drugs and asthma 155
Dry air 64
Dry cleaning 246
Dull ache 81
Dust 226
Dust mites 107, 227

E

Ear ache 283
Earplanes 25
Ears 22
Echinacea extract 197
Elimination diet 215
Enlarged prostate and antihistamines 132
Epinephrine 155
Essential oils 289
Ethmoid sinus 6, 7
    infection 82
Ethmoidectomy 140
Eustachian tube 23
Exercise 214, 220
    illness and 198
Expectorant 161, 179, 283
    herbal 200
External nares 9

F

Facial pain 82
Faith and healing 270
Fatigue 83, 243
Fel d1 107
Feldenkrais 267
Fenugreek 240
Fever 84, 283

Fish oils 214
Flower essences 288
Flu 37, 39
Folk remedies 239
Food allergy 109
Free radicals 203
Frontal sinus 6, 7
    infection 82

G

Garlic 242
Gas stoves and asthma 152
Ginkgo biloba 240
Guided imagery 261

H

Hatha yoga 259
Hayfever 283
Hazardous occupations 74
Head congestion 81
Headache 46, 81, 244
Helicobacter pylori 166
Herbal sleep formulas 196
Herbal tea 200, 219
Herbalism 280
Herbs 205
    contraindications 284
    list of 282
High efficiency particulate
    arrestor 232
Histamine 66
Hoarseness 84
Holistic medicine 251
Home air purifiers 152
Homeopathy 284
Honey 240
Horseradish 243
Hot beverages 242
Household plants 234
Hydration 133
    athsma 143

Hydrocarbon 58
Hygiene 188
Hypnotherapy 259

I

Ice 241
Immune bodies 33
Immune support 283
Immune system
   antibiotics 125
   187
   stress 223
Immunity 31
Industrial exhaust 112
Infectants 165, 167
Ingestants 165, 167
Inhalants 165, 167
Injectants 165, 167
Internal nares 9
Ion imbalance 62
Isoproterenol 155

J

Japanese green tea 206

L

Laryngitis 21, 84
Laryngopharynx 18
Larynx 19
Lemon peel 240

M

Massage therapy 267
Maxillary sinus 6, 7
   infection 82
   toothache 47
Meditation 266, 273
Melatonin 196
Methylxanthine 156

Mold 107, 229
Moxibustion 277
Mucous mem-
   brane 12, 51, 87, 200
Mucus production 84

N

Nasal congestion 84
Nasal decongestant sprays 129
Nasal irrigation 176
Naso-antral window 140
Nasopharynx 18
Natural immunity 33
Naturopathic medicine 264
Negative ions 233
Neuralgia of the trigeminal
   nerve 46
Nicotine 50, 190
Nitrogen dioxide 152
Nitrogen oxide 57
Nose 8
   function 10
   structure 11
Nose blowing 242
Nostrils 9

O

Omega-3 fatty acids 214
Oropharynx 18
Osteopathic medicine 263
Ostia 3
Otitis media and children 26
   food allergy 27
Otolaryngoly evaluation 138
Oxidation 204
Ozone 58

P

Pain 283
Pain relievers and children 133

Paranasal sinuses 6
Parasitic worms and allergy 166
Peace of mind 268
Peak-flow meters 162
Perfume 247
Pesticides 112
Pets 107
Pharynx 16
Physical stress 222
Phytochemicals 207
Pollen 106, 173, 230
Pollutants 61
  indoor 231
Pollution 55, 57
Polyp 76
Postural drainage 181
Pregnancy and asthma 169
Psychological stress 222
Psychotherapy 261
Pulmonary function test 148

R

Radio nuclides 62
Radon 62, 115, 234
Recovery tonics 283
Reflexology 275, 293
Relaxation 263
Religious faith 272
Respiratory 283
Rest 194, 218
Rhinitis 44, 283
  allergic 106
Rolfing 267
Runny nose 244

S

Saline irrigation 134
Saline spray 134
Salt water 241
Secondhand smoke 51, 52, 111,
  191

dietary help 192
Selenium 205
Self Care Catalogue 151
Shiatsu 268
Sick Building Syndrome 62, 97
Sinobronchitis 110, 180
Sinus
  definition 3
  descripton 3
  functions 4
Sinus irrigation 218
Sinusitis 80
  acute 43, 88, 119
  asthma 98
  causes 42, 48
  children 44, 82
  chronic 43, 85, 90
  description 41
  definition 8
  diagnosis 44, 76
  essential oils first aid kit 292
  flower essence first aid
    kit 286
  herbal first aid kit 284
  homeopathic first aid kit 285
  treatment 47
Sleep 195
  cellular damage 220
Sleeping 246
Smell, sense of 13
Smoke 51
Smoking 190
Sore throat 244, 283
Sphenoid sinus 6, 8
  infection 82
Spicy foods 242
Status asthmaticus 103
Steam 241
Stress 221, 258
  asthma 105
  management 223
  vitamins 200

Stuffy nose 244
Sulfur dioxide 57, 116
Surfer's ear 31
Swimmer's ear 30

T

Taste, sense of 15
Temporal arteritis 46
Theophylline 156
Throat, irritated 84
Thymus 35, 245
Toilet paper 247
Toothache 46
  maxillary sinus 47
Traditional Chinese medi-
  cine 279
Trager 268
Tumors 47
Tympanostomy 29

V

Vacuum cleaners, anti-
  allergen 173
Valerian 197
Vaporizer, ultrasonic 134
Viruses and asthma 98
Visualization 261
Vitamin C 198

W

Water 216
Wheezing 245
Women and asthma 152

Y

Yeast 236
Yeast infection 237
Yoga 259

Z

Zinc extract drops 198